Belief, Mystery, Miracles, and Eternity:

WHERE SCIENCE AND SPIRITUALITY CAN AGREE

John K. Graham, M.D., Ph.D., D.Min.

Printed in the United States of America
First Edition

Library of Congress Cataloging-in-Publication Data
Belief, Mystery, Miracles, and Eternity: Where Science and Spirituality Can Agree
by Graham, John K

All-Reality Press
Bellaire, TX 77401
www.all-reality.org

Key Words: Science Spirituality Quantum Physics Metaphysics Creation Reality Consciousness Religion Holographic Intelligent Universe

ISBN 979-8-9990380-1-2 (eBook)
ISBN 979-8-9990380-0-5 (Paperback)

V10152025

This book is dedicated with love to my dear wife
Patsy "Pat" Stamps Graham
who has been my companion in life, my best friend, and has faithfully supported me no matter the sacrifice required.
And she gave us five wonderful children.

This book is dedicated with love to my [illegible]

[illegible]

Endorsements

"Dr John Graham is a scientist, scholar and life-long practitioner equally of faith and medicine. What makes Dr Graham and his message essential, is that he unveils the profound sacredness, the very presence of G-d, in every bit of life, including as perceived through science. People of faith can know that science is a form of witness, just as we give testimony one by one, we can look at the chorus of human experience in a study sample. Graham is 100% doctor and 100% faithful!"

Dr. Lisa Miller, Professor, Columbia University and Author, *The Awakened Brain; The New Science of Spirituality and Our Quest for an Inspired Life*. Founder, Spirituality Mind Body Institute.

"John Graham is a physician who deploys the insights and tools of science to heal while recognizing his patients are spiritual animals who exceed what science can tell. He is a student who brings to bear science, clinical experience, and spiritual traditions to grapple with the mysteries of the human condition. Join him on a journey into the deep questions raised by science and spirituality."

Farr Curlin, M.D., Josiah C Trent Professor of Medical Humanities | Professor of Medicine | Co-Director, Theology, Medicine, and Culture Initiative | Duke University

---

"A profound contribution! A book for those who wonder at the world, who search for answers to bewildering questions, who struggle to find a greater purpose, who look for reasons to be hopeful, and who seek a deeper dimension in life. With wisdom gleaned from up-to-date science, the world's great religious traditions, and his own remarkable life journey, John Graham explores topics often neglected, but vital to what it means to be fully human. Here we read about mystery, miracles, suffering, evil, consciousness, the possibility of life after death, and the sacred. Graham sees each of these topics through multiple lenses, but is able to create a unifying vision, one that provides a space for both "reason and reverence." For all of its great breadth and depth, this is a very readable book filled with the warmth, wonder, hopefulness, and insatiable curiosity of the author. It should be read by scientists, religious and spiritual people, and anyone interested in finding greater wholeness in a time of brokenness."

Kenneth Pargament, Ph.D., Distinguished Scholar, Professor of Psychology, author of *Spiritually Integrated Psychotherapy: Understanding and Addressing the Sacred; The Psychology of Religion and Coping*.

"This comprehensive synthesis of modern science and spirituality provides a practical guide to strengthening beliefs in a benevolent force in the universe, embracing life's mysteries and appreciating our connection to miracles and eternity. With lifelong experience as a physician and preacher, Dr. Graham shares his illuminated observations to offer a harmonious world view, especially useful in these confused times."

Eben Alexander, M.D., Former Harvard Neurosurgeon and author of *Proof of Heaven, The Map of Heaven, and Living in a Mindful Universe*

"In asking the foundational questions of the how and why of our existence, science and spirituality are John K Graham's companions in his quest for truth. Sharing his profound and powerful journey of inner and outer discovery; to 'begin with mystery and end with love' is perhaps the greatest gift and ultimate homecoming that their convergence and resolution offer us. Together they reveal who we really are, as microcosmic co-creators of our Universe's ineffable wonder, and who we can evolve to become."

Dr. Jude Currivan, Cosmologist and author of *The Cosmic Hologram* and co-founder of WholeWorld-View: www.wholeworld-view.org

---

"With the wisdom of a healer and the heart of a seeker, Belief, Mystery, Miracles, and Eternity invites readers into a conversation that is both intellectually rich and spiritually nourishing. Written for those yearning to live with both reason and reverence, Dr. Graham reminds us that spirituality is not an escape from science, but a deeper journey into what it means to be fully human."

Nathan Carlin, Ph.D., Director of the McGovern Center for Humanities and Ethics and author of *Pastoral Aesthetics: A Theological Perspective on Principlist Bioethics*

"Belief, Mystery, Miracles, and Eternity invites readers into a thin space where scalpels and sacraments, PET scans and psalms, enter dialogue without dissonance. Dr. John K. Graham—surgeon, priest, and seeker—writes with the knowledge, wisdom, and warmth of Eucharistic, showing how "belief is not just a private emotion but a powerful force shaping body, brain, and soul". From near-death encounters in the OR to quantum hints of a conscious cosmos, he gathers neuroscience, contemplative practice, and lived stories of hope into a single, luminous arc. The result is a field guide for anyone who has ever wondered whether intellect and intimacy with God can live under one roof.

"Graham's vision also echoes a distinctly Anglican confidence that mystery deepens, rather than diminishes, the mind. As Sir Thomas Browne, the seventeenth-century physician-theologian, marveled, "I love to lose myself in a mystery, to pursue my reason to an O altitudo!" Following that spirit, Graham shows that miracles can be portals instead of puzzle-pieces, that eternity can be embraced without abandoning empiricism, and that loving inquiry—into cells, stars, or scripture—may itself be the greatest act of faith. Vivid, rigorous, and pastoral, this book doesn't merely bridge the gap between science and spirituality; it invites readers to walk across the abyss."

C. Andrew Doyle, is the IX Bishop of the Episcopal Diocese of Texas, and author of *Unabashed Faith*, 2025.

"John Graham's groundbreaking work on spiritual health is a powerful continuation of tradition. His insights echo the visionary stance taken by Swiss Federal Councilor Philipp Etter at the inaugural World Health Assembly in 1948, where the term "spiritual" was first introduced into the global health conversation. Etter's call for a holistic understanding of health—one that includes the spiritual dimension—laid the foundation for decades of debate and development within the WHO. Graham builds on this legacy with clarity and conviction, offering a compelling framework that bridges medicine, ministry, and meaning. His book doesn't just revisit old ideas, it revitalizes them, proving their enduring relevance in today's fractured healthcare landscape. In a world hungry for healing that transcends the physical, Graham's voice is both timely and timeless. This is more than a book, it's a call to remember what health was always meant to be: whole."

Dr. Derek Yach, MBChB, MPH, DSc, Global health advocate, researcher, and policy maker formerly at WHO, Yale, Rockefeller Foundation. Currently, focus is on the role of faith-based health groups in health and the need to incorporate spirituality dimensions in health policies.

"With fresh insight, Dr. John Graham invites us to explore the human experience—a tapestry woven with mystery, awe, the miraculous, as well as the spiritual and faith dimension of the worship of God. Merging thousands of years of spiritual and religious tradition with the emerging science of a fine-turned, Intelligent and Conscious Universe (God), Graham offers a compelling new vision. I highly recommend this book to anyone ready to move beyond materialism to embrace what Graham describes as a Theory of Reality (TOR)—a unifying framework that integrates both scientific understanding and spiritual truth, under the overarching love of God."

Harold G. Koenig, M.D., M.H.Sc.
Professor of Psychiatry and Behavioral Sciences, Associate Professor of Medicine
Duke University Medical Center, Durham, North Carolina
Adjunct Professor, Department of Medicine, King Abdulaziz University, Saudi Arabia
Visiting Professor, Shiraz University of Medical Sciences, Shiraz, Iran
Editor-in-Chief, International Journal of Psychiatry in Medicine
https://spiritualityandhealth.duke.edu/index.php/harold-g-koenig-m-d/

"In these 21st century times of accelerating conflict and even violence, it will become more important than ever to seek innovative solutions for addressing internal and global tensions. This must include efforts to bridge an expanding divide between science and religion. Too often such differences are viewed as inherent and blamed for extreme divisiveness around important societal issues in modern medicine and public health, including vaccinations, bioinformatics and gene therapies, and climate health, to name a few.

"The Jesuit priest and paleontologist Dr. Pierre Teilhard de Chardin once famously wrote: "After close on two centuries of passionate struggles, neither science nor faith has succeeded in discrediting its adversary," but even now reconciling these two forces remains elusive.

"Towards that goal, in his new book, Belief, Mystery, Miracles, and Eternity, the Texas Medical Center physician and Episcopal priest, Dr. John K. Graham explains how science and spirituality can indeed find common ground. In so doing, Dr. Graham provides us with a roadmap for closing the gaps between science and religion as an essential step towards acceptance and collaboration."

Peter Hotez M.D., Ph.D.
Professor of Pediatric and Molecular Virology
Dean, National School of Tropical Medicine
Baylor College of Medicine in the Texas Medical Center
by Hotez: *The Deadly Rise of Anti-Science; Vaccines Did Not Cause Rachel's Autism; Forgotten People, Forgotten Diseases; Blue Marble Health: An Innovative Plan to Fight Diseases of the Poor Amid Wealth*

"John Graham is an Episcopal priest and surgeon, who earned a doctorate in mind-body medicine. He is uniquely qualified to bridge the gap between science and spirituality. He invites us to share his own path of exploration, that has brought him to see the world with new eyes and an open heart. Graham draws on the latest reports from neuroscience, neurobiology, and the science of consciousness, as well as the wisdom of the Buddha, St. Augustine, and Carl Jung, to illuminate his search for the meeting point of science and spiritual awakening. I recommend this very personal text, that guides us from cell biology to the recognition of "love as the final word.""

Donald Moss, Ph.D., Professor and Dean, College of Integrative Medicine and Health Sciences, Saybrook University, Pasadena, CA. By Moss: *Humanistic and Transpersonal Psychology: A Historical and Biographical Sourcebook; Phenomenology, Applied Psychophysiology, and Behavioral Medicine; Alzheimer's: My Journey to a Next Generation Treatment*

"In Belief, Mystery, Miracles, and Eternity, Dr. John K. Graham masterfully weaves science and spirituality into a tapestry of hope, awe, and transformation. His profound reflections invite readers to embrace the wonder of the field of infinite potential and evolving intelligence, experience divine presence and ancient wisdom, and discover the miracle of cosmic order in the universe and within every cell in our bodies. Dr. Graham's masterpiece is a harmonious blend of scientific rigor and spiritual depth, revealing the beauty of our interconnected universe and the depths of human experience. You will be challenged, affirmed, and blessed."

The Reverend Gena Davis, Episcopal Priest, Spiritual Director, Author, Healing Arts Practitioner, and Founder of YogaMass, Inc.

"In this monumental work, Dr. John K. Graham explores the most important and timeless questions we can ask as human beings. His reflections, from scientific exposition to personal storytelling, provoke inspiration, wonder, and a sense of awe at how far we have come, and how far we've yet to go. This book is a journey into the deepest aspects of reality, guided by a brilliant thinker whose life of faithful learning, teaching, healing, guiding, and growing, positions him uniquely to accompany us."

Stuart A. Nelson, M.A., President, Institute for Spirituality and Health.

"In this most recent of Dr. John Graham's gifts to us he coveys how the concept of CALLING transforms occupations into Sacred Vocations that lead one to give to others as one feels BLESSED to have received from a Higher Power. He tells meaningful stories of times when he felt challenged and inadequate, but overcame deficiencies which seemed insurmountable because of a loving, transcendent gift or gifts from his God. Each time he then felt and acted upon a Calling to give to others his version of what he could offer at different moments in his life: extraordinary medical care, pastoral guidance, and then educational experiences about the synergy, not divergence of science and faith. Readers will benefit from his sharing disclosures about his imperfections and the value of HOPE in the midst of uncertainty and threat. While this gift would be a treasure at any time, it is a particular value at this time of so much divisive polarization being exploited by so many malevolent leaders."

James W. Lomax, M.D. - Emeritus Professor of Psychiatry, former Karl Menninger Chair of Psychiatric Education, Menninger Department of Psychiatry and Behavioral Sciences, Baylor College of Medicine, Houston, TX. He is also a former president of the American Association of Directors of Psychiatry Residency Training (AADPRT), Fellow of the American College of Psychiatrists (ACP), and Distinguished Fellow of the American Psychiatric Association (APA).

Contents

Preface: An Invitation to Wonder

In life, what divides families, friends, and colleagues is often the facts we embrace as ultimate truth. This is also true for the separation that exists between science and spirituality. But, what if the mysteries that have inspired saints, seekers, and sages for thousands of years, are now found in the very language of quantum physics and sub-atomic particles in modern science?

In recent years, science—particularly physics—has begun to explore astonishing ideas. That consciousness might not arise from the brain but be woven into the very fabric of the universe. That everything and everyone is interconnected. That death may not be the final chapter. That what we call "miracles" might not violate the laws of physical nature but instead may reveal a higher natural order we are just beginning to perceive.

The era of materialism's dominance is fading (Menuge, 2023). We have now entered the era of post-materialism where an affirmation of spiritual truths humanity has long revered—belief in the soul, the miraculous, and life after death—are glimpses that embrace a deeper, quantum reality. This is the foundation for what I cultivate in this book—to find where science and spirituality can agree.

And, if these two radically different disciples can find agreement, so can all that divides.

Whether science and spirituality can be united is not theoretical—for me, it has been my lived experience. I have walked in a white coat. I have worn clerical robes. I have lived in both worlds. Science and spirituality. Science embraces **the what**; spirituality embraces **the why**. I love both.

And—we need both.

I began my professional life engaged in the rigor of the physical sciences. After graduating from Tulane Medical School, I pursued a career in medicine, embracing the sharp delineation between science and spirituality that so many in science accept without question. The two domains, I believed, were fundamentally separate—perhaps irreconcilable.

But then, at the age of 35, a spiritual experience shattered that divide for me. It was an encounter so profound that I could no longer cling to the belief that the physical world was all there is. The impact of that experience inspired me to become an Episcopal priest and to write this book to share how we can find a place of agreement even where it seems impossible. In the Appendix to this book, I have included a description of four encounters with God. I encourage reading that section to understand how I felt called to leave medicine to become an Episcopal priest.

Belief, Mystery, Miracles, and Eternity, is an invitation to look again—to see with new eyes and an open heart. It is written for the seekers and the skeptics alike, for those who suspect that life holds more meaning, more mystery, and more connection than we have been taught to believe.

Our journey begins with belief—because revisiting our core beliefs (the facts) can open the door to transformation and wonder, and wonder is the first step to find wisdom that unites.

For centuries, since the days of Descartes, we have lived with a split—a great division between body and soul, science and spirit. But that division is beginning to heal. Quantum science shows us that all things are connected—that we live not in a universe of separation, but of deep and mysterious unity. Ecumenical teacher and Franciscan priest, Richard Rohr (2016), has said,

> Right now, we are finding quantum physics, biology, and cosmology are finally at a level of development that our understanding of everything from atoms to galaxies to organisms is affirming, confirming, and allowing us to use

> old faith language and right now with a new level of appreciation.
>
> Now is the right time—the critical time—to explore all that divides, not with a sword, but with the heartfelt desire to bring us together.

My life changed radically following my spiritually-awakening experience. In the applied science of medicine, as a plastic and reconstructive surgeon, I had many opportunities to serve people in their hour of great need. One involved a four-year-old boy, Robert, whose arm had been totally amputated above the elbow on the back of a farm tractor. Using the training I had received in microsurgery and in reconstructive plastic surgery I was able to replant his arm on "Good Friday," April 7, 1977. Years later he was able to pass a physical exam to become an FBI agent. Another young boy, Chad, sustained a shotgun blast to his face that ripped his face apart. In the operating room, working with an oral surgeon, we were able to rebuild the child's face. Years later, Chad graduated from medical school and today is an anesthesiologist.

After serving for 15 years as a practicing physician, I felt called to the ministry. I attended the Episcopal Seminary of the Southwest and served in churches in Austin and Houston for 20 years. In 2010, I became President and CEO of the Institute for Spirituality and Health at the Texas Medical Center, in Houston (ISH).

This brought together my experience as a physician and as a priest which allowed me to embrace a great divide and to love both—science (the physical universe) and spirituality (the metaphysical dimension)—which together embrace the whole of the human experience as we know it.

I will not argue that science and spirituality must be blended in order to be united. They are different disciplines, and rightly so. Each offers a vital way of seeing. Each points to truth. Each addresses the mystery and calls us to wonder. Each gives us the opportunity to discover how to embrace both without losing either.

That is the key.

This book is my humble offering. A weaving together of belief and mystery, miracle and eternity, science and spirituality, head and heart. Above all it is a witness to wholeness that is already present—waiting to be revealed in science and spirituality, and in all of life.

Before Proceeding

First, although this book is written from my own spiritual perspective, I believe it will also be recognized that I have made a heart-felt effort to affirm people of all faiths because I have seen God's love and grace is present in everyone. And, because of the discoveries in quantum physics, I know we are all **interconnected** whether we know it or not. We are one with The Source, God.

Second, I make every effort in my book to document the discoveries of science as well as to affirm the spiritual experiences that I and countless others cannot deny. For me, both the material universe and the spiritual dimension must be valued, respected and affirmed. The material universe is a gift; and the spiritual dimension is a gift.

Third, I believe the discoveries of quantum physics affirm both the material and spiritual dimensions of reality. Although the long-awaited Theory of Everything (TOE) in physics refers to the union of classical and quantum physics; for me, when science and the metaphysical come together, they inform what could become an ultimate, unified, singular, all-encompassing, coherent Theory of Reality (TOR) that unites all humanity experiences as reality.

Join me now as we look at *Belief, Mystery, Miracles, and Eternity: Where Science and Spirituality Can Agree*.

Below is a prayer I was taught by my friend, Lex Gillan, at our Institute in his yoga training class. It is my prayer as I seek wisdom that unites. Perhaps, it can be your prayer, as well.

Truth, awaken in me (Anonymous)

Illuminate me with Your presence.
Shine Your light into all the dark places.
Reveal to me Your understanding.
Shower me with the light of Your peace.
Move me closer in passionate inspiration.
Uplift my being with Your radiant joy.

Infuse my body with Your healing light.
Infuse my mind with the light of wisdom.
Infuse my heart with creative passion.
Infuse my spirit with loving-kindness.
Truth, come alive within me.
Set me free in You.

PART I: BELIEF

Introduction to Part I, Belief

When someone is asked why they hold a particular belief to be true, most will hesitate and say, "I never really thought about it."

Yet what we believe and how we arrive at our beliefs is of importance when we consider the deep issues in life such as mystery, miracles, eternity, and whether there is life after death. Then too, we have beliefs about almost everything, and we also have what are called our core beliefs and values. Core beliefs are fundamental convictions that guide our behavior and thought processes. Identifying these is important for personal growth and self-awareness. Throughout this chapter you may have questions arise that invite you to ponder your beliefs and ask yourself, "What do I truly value?", "What influences my beliefs?", or "How do I respond to challenges?" Asking these kinds of questions can help uncover our core beliefs.

How do we arrive at our beliefs? What does science and spirituality have to offer? To answer these questions, we begin our study exploring the nature, sources, and transformative power of belief in our life.

As we ponder the power of belief together, recall this well-known statement attributed to 6th Century B.C., Taoist philosopher, Lao Tzu: "Watch your thoughts, they become your words; watch your words, they become your actions; watch your actions, they become your habits; watch your habits, they become your character; watch your character, it becomes your destiny."

When I look back over my own life, I can see how many times my personal beliefs have shifted and deepened. In the preface, I mentioned the story of my spiritual awakening that changed everything. But that is only one of many transformations to be explored.

On Religion

And an old priest said, Speak to us of Religion. And he said:
Have I spoken this day of aught else?
Is not religion all deeds and all reflection,
And that which is neither deed nor reflection,
but a wonder and a surprise ever springing in the soul,
even while the hand hew the stone or tend the loom?
Who can separate his faith from his actions, or his belief from his occupations?
Who can spread his hours before him, saying, "This for God and this for myself'
This for my soul, and this other for my body?"
And if you would know God be not therefore a solver of riddles.
Rather look about you and you shall see Him playing with your children.
And look into space; you shall see Him walking on beams of light,
outstretching His arms in the lightning and descending in rain.
You shall see Him smiling in flowers, then rising and waving His hands in trees.

Public Domain Poem, by Kahlil Gibran (1883-1931)

Chapter 1—Belief Defined

Why begin with a section on belief? Because belief is the invisible architecture of our lives. It frames how we see the world, how we understand ourselves, and how we dare to dream beyond what is visible. Whether we believe in a spiritual dimension that pulses beneath the surface of things or affirm—like many devoted scientists—that only the material universe is real, our beliefs hold power. They govern our thoughts, our choices, and even our openness to mystery.

Yet when our beliefs are questioned, we can feel threatened. Our first instinct is often to defend rather than to reflect, to shield rather than to wonder. But what we need is to be aware. Awareness is the key.

Before we journey into the vast landscapes of Mystery, Miracles, and Eternity, it is wise to pause and ask: *What do I believe?* And perhaps more importantly: *Am I willing to acknowledge there may be things I can see anew?*

Only with an open mind—and a willing heart—can we begin to explore what lies beyond the familiar horizon.

What is belief?

Harvard psychologist William James said belief is a perception of reality (James, 1889). While that is true, the common understanding is that belief is an affirmation we hold that something is true or real—even without definitive proof. For example, we might say, "She believes her hard work will be rewarded." Time will reveal whether her belief was well-founded. Belief can also express trust or faith in someone or something: "He trusts in God," or "I have faith in the findings of science."

It's sobering to realize that we can have a long-held belief—one that affects how we treat ourselves or others—even if it has no foundation in fact.

For example, Dr. Victor Oboli (2025) shared in *JAMA* that a 5-year-old critically injured child was rushed into his emergency room at Yale School of Medicine and died a short time later despite all their efforts to save her. Upon learning her daughter had died, the child's mother became hysterical, slapped Dr. Oboli across the face, and said, "You killed my only daughter!" Several weeks later she returned to the hospital, met with Dr. Oboli and apologized for falsely accusing him of having killed her daughter.

In the bereavement support group that I facilitate, I have heard bereaved individuals blame others for their loved one's death—the ambulance driver was too slow, my husband refused to go for an fMRI, or that their doctor missed the diagnosis. After emotions have subsided, they seldom mention it again.

There is also a difference between belief and knowledge. Knowledge is a belief that is justified because there is evidence to support that belief. Yet, beliefs are not simply passive recipients of information; rather, our brain actively processes the data we perceive through our five senses followed by assessment of that data before we arrive at and espouse our beliefs.

David Hume (1711-1776) contributed greatly to our understanding that belief can be with or without factual knowledge and in a book published after his death Hume states, "A wise man proportions the strength of his beliefs based on the evidence" (Hume, 1977).

Science and Belief

In science, belief is built slowly—through observation, experimentation, and cautious interpretation. Research protocols are known to be subject to bias, flawed design, lack of generalizability, and ethical concerns, to name only a few limitations. For this reason, following publication of results, replication by other researchers is required to verify findings.

Interestingly, scientists often begin by proposing a **"null hypothesis,"** a negative statement they hope to disprove (Hagen, 1997). For example: "This treatment has no effect on headache relief." If evidence disproves the statement, scientists can support a new belief: that the treatment likely does help. Still, such conclusions are never absolute. Science always leaves room for doubt, error, and the need for replication. That humility is its strength.

In the world of quantum physics, uncertainty is not a flaw—it is woven into the very fabric of reality. Werner Heisenberg's **Uncertainty or Indeterminacy Principle** shows that there is a fundamental limit to knowing both the position and the momentum of a quantum particle at the same time. This is not due to human error, but to the nature of existence itself.

Similarly, when we reflect on our own beliefs, it is wise to recognize that, however much evidence or knowledge we gather, a measure of **uncertainty remains**—and perhaps must remain. It is this humility that keeps us seeking, growing, and reaching ever closer to the truth that lies beyond full human comprehension.

On Certainty

The careful, methodical approach of science reminds us to approach our personal beliefs with the same thoughtfulness and humility. In both science and spirituality, certainty can be the enemy of truth.

Even the brilliant Albert Einstein was not immune to error. In developing his general theory of relativity, Einstein introduced a "cosmological constant" so his equations would fit what he believed—that our universe was a static universe.

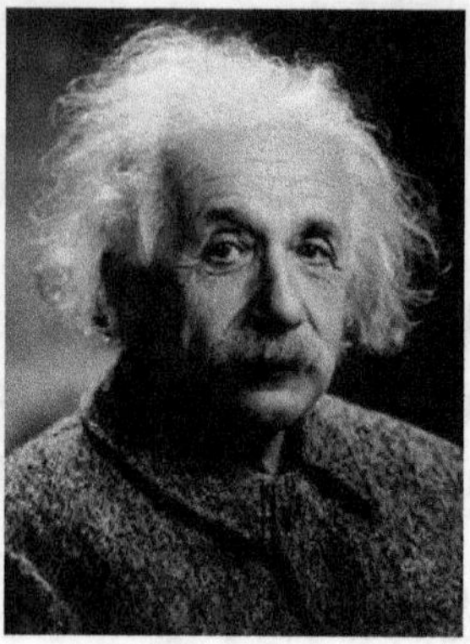

Albert Einstein, Public Domain, Wikimedia Commons. Original image source: http://www.loc.gov/rr/print/list/235_poe.html. U.S. Library of Congress - Famous People]. Photograph by Oren Jack Turner, Princeton, N.J. Copyrighted 1947, Not renewed. Reproduction Number LC-USZ62-

Years later, when discoveries revealed the universe is not static but rapidly expanding, Einstein called this "adjustment" (adding a cosmological constant) the greatest blunder of his career. If a mind like Einstein's can err, so can we. His story reminds us why science cultivates a healthy measure of skepticism—a humility before the unknown.

Cognitively, we humans seek the answer to any controversial issue that may arise. It appears we often already have our mind made up and search for someone "in authority" who will express what we want to hear. Unwisely, we may embrace answers proposed by almost any religious, societal, psychological, economic, or political leader even though the issue is not within their area of expertise. For example, a physicist's judgement of spiritual matters, and conversely, a pastor rejecting scientific findings. Both views should be suspect. Today, we are able to share misinformation with others over social media, and they share the same misinformation with countless others who may accept online postings as factual. In reality, we may well be sharing a myth which can be lethal as with the antivaccination movement.

The Antivaccine Movement and Misinformation

The antivaccine movement in the United States and Europe is a classic example of a belief that affects the lives of children yet has no foundation in fact. Vaccination is often proclaimed on social media as the cause of autism although many research studies have consistently shown there is no correlation. In the 1990s, Andrew Wakefield, a London physician published an article claiming to have found, in eight patients, the explanation for autism in the measles vaccine. Although the article was immediately repudiated by neurologists, this did not stop the media and autism support groups from spreading misinformation. In a revealing article, Neurologist Michael Davidson, M.D. shares how the search for an answer can blind us to truth. He writes:

> Wakefield's findings should have looked highly suspicious. Anybody who has ever been around autistic children and observed how phenomenologically diverse they are would have doubted that the biological underpinning of the condition affecting all eight subjects could be the same. Doubts aside, the measles vaccine hypothesis had all the ingredients necessary to become, nearly overnight, the accepted wisdom (for a full explanation, I recommend reading this review found in References: Davidson, 2017).

From the department of Pediatrics and Molecular virology and Microbiology at the Baylor College of Medicine, Olive et al. (2018), have addressed the movement that has encouraged parents to take a "philosophical" or "religious belief" exemption to vaccinating their children. The tragedy is that unvaccinated children are 35 times more likely to contact measles than a vaccinated child. And a child without the Diphtheria, tetanus, and pertussis (DTaP) vaccine is three times more likely to contact pertussis than a vaccinated child. Furthermore, the antivaccine movement has weakened "herd immunity" that protects the population at large and especially provides protection to children who cannot be vaccinated for medical reasons.

Highlighting the seriousness of what has become a global health issue, Baylor College of Medicine's, Dr. Peter Hotez (2019), has authored an article entitled, *America and Europe's New Normal: The Return of Vaccine Preventable Diseases*, in which he has documented the dramatic rise in the unvaccinated diseases that can be lethal, including measles, pertussis, influenza, and human papillomavirus, a cause of cervical cancer in women. As far as vaccination being the cause of autism in children, Hotez states studies have now found changes occur in the brain prior to birth, long before a child has been immunized. Scientific studies have also found genetic changes in as many as 99 genes associated with autism.

The reality is misinformation has the power to influence behavior in parents that can put the life of their children at risk. As stated previously, it is important to consider the source of our beliefs, and it is wise to hold a measure of doubt where there is controversy.

Religious Beliefs Matter

No exploration of belief would be complete without opening the door to assess religious faith—that ancient, enduring pathway by which humanity seeks the sacred. Across time and culture, religious beliefs have provided comfort, helping countless souls navigate life's mysteries. Yet, Balboni et al. (2022) write that, "despite growing evidence, the role of spirituality in serious illness and health has not been systematically assessed." Awareness of the gap in recognition of the role spirituality plays in health care is important when extensive research has revealed the depth spirituality and religious beliefs play in the lives of patients (Koenig et al., 2023).

A recent survey of 11,201 U.S. adults (Pew Research Center, 2023) reveals that even in our modern age, belief in the divine remains widespread. Fully 83% of adults believe people have a soul or spirit in addition to their physical body. 81% say there is something spiritual beyond the natural world, even if they cannot see it. 74% say there are some things that science cannot possibly explain. 38% say they have had a strong feeling that someone who has passed away was communicating with them from beyond this world. And, overall, 70% of U.S. adults say they can be considered "spiritual" in some way, because they think of themselves as spiritual people or say spirituality is very important in their lives. 30% say they have personally encountered a spirit or unseen spiritual force and profess belief in God or a higher power.

Furthermore, 90% of U.S. adults believe in God or another higher power, while only 10% do not. Yet, the nature of that belief is as varied: only 54% affirm the God described in the Bible, while another 34% don't believe in the biblical God but do believe there is some higher power or spiritual force in the universe, something sacred, vast, and alive beyond themselves. 71% believe in heaven and, perhaps surprisingly, 61% believe in hell, while over 50% believe it is "probably" or "definitely" true that the deceased can be reunited with loved ones who died prior to them.

Nearly half of Americans believe that God or a higher power directly shapes the events of their lives "all or most of the time," and another 18% feel this divine hand "some of the time." Eight in ten adults speak of being protected by God, and two-thirds tell stories of blessings they attribute to a higher Presence. Three-quarters say they regularly talk to God—and three in ten hear God speaking back.

Among Christians, belief in the biblical God remains especially strong: 80% affirm this is their belief, while another 19% describe their trust in broader spiritual terms. Only a small fraction—1%—have no belief in any higher power. Jewish Americans and religious "nones" are more likely to hold non-traditional views, yet even among these groups, the yearning for the divine persists. The majority—89% of Jews and 72% of unaffiliated individuals—profess belief in a spiritual force or presence, even if they do not envision the God of the Bible.

Although there were too few Muslim, Hindu, Buddhist, and other minority religious voices in the Pew study to draw firm conclusions, their presence in America's spiritual tapestry continues to grow, offering many and varied perceptions of the divine.

Religion's Unique Focus

Psychologist Kenneth Pargament and his colleagues (2005) state that religious belief is uniquely defined by its focus on the sacred—a central reality from which meaning, morality, and motivation flow. Unlike other beliefs, religious faith touches every dimension of the human spirit: it offers strength in times of suffering, in seasons of doubt, and hope when facing despair.

The journey of faith often begins early and is perhaps motivated in a child's longing for parental approval or fear of divine punishment. In adulthood, it evolves into a search for community, for belonging, and for significance. For many, it becomes a lifelong pilgrimage toward the heart of the sacred—a search not for approval or status, but for meaning, purpose, and divine love.

The fruits of religious belief are profound. Research shows that those who nurture a strong relationship with God or a higher power report greater satisfaction with life, lower levels of depression, and deeper bonds within marriage (Koenig et al., 2023). In the end, religious belief may offer more than comfort—it may weave a sense of coherence through the soul, binding together heart, mind, and spirit in a living tapestry of hope, resilience, and meaning.

In the realm of spirituality, questions and doubt should not be seen as threats to one's faith; instead, they can be partners in its growth.

When individuals or religious communities claim absolute certainty about the nature of the divine, spiritual life can become stagnant and rigid. Those with differing perspectives may be labeled as misguided or dangerous. Over time, this attitude of certainty can lead to isolation, exclusion, and a loss of the dynamic openness that is required to experience spiritual vitality.

It is easy to forget that the sacred texts of our faith were written by inspired individuals, but human beings nonetheless—people shaped by the language, culture, and understanding of their own time. When scripture is viewed as literally the word of God, it can, ironically, miss the living reality of the God it seeks to reveal. Conversely, experiencing the reality of the living God can challenge the interpretation of scripture and long held beliefs.

Furthermore, cultivating relationships with those of different traditions can deepen our encounter with the Sacred. It can expand our vision of a loving deity who transcends human boundaries and welcomes the marginalized, the outcast, and those we previously considered unacceptable. It is wise to ponder who were—and are now—considered unacceptable.

Scientific Beliefs Matter

Columbia University Professor of Psychology and associates, Miller, L. et al. (2019), used fMRI recordings and self-reported data from a diverse group of participants to study the neural mechanisms of personally meaningful spiritual experiences when compared to stressful or neutral, relaxing experiences. The study found that strong spiritual states are associated with a sense of connection to someone or something greater than oneself such as a higher power, God, or transcendent figure or consciousness. Subjects also reported a perceived oneness and dissolution of the boundary between self and others. Although a spiritual experience can occur at any time, study participants reported the experience occurring when engaged in mindfulness meditation and prayer, when out-of-doors in nature, and when participating in worship within a religious community.

The authors concluded that study findings demonstrated neural mechanisms mediated by the brain are associated with spiritual experiences across diverse religious and cultural perspectives.

The Awakened Brain

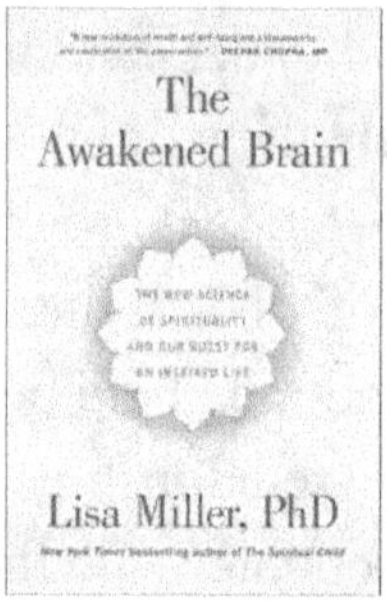

In her book, *The Awakened Brain: The New Science of Spirituality and Our Quest for an Inspired Life* (2021), Columbia University Teacher College, Professor of Psychology, Lisa Miller reports a long-term data analysis to examine the relationship between spirituality and depression for early adults aged sixteen to twenty-six. Participants in the study had a high familial risk for depression and had grown up in a household where depression was ever-present. Two findings emerged in this study: First, those who had a strong personal spirituality at age twenty-six were two and a half times more likely to have been depressed in the past. Meaning, spiritual maturity developed alongside or through their struggles. Second, those who had strong spirituality by age twenty-six were 75 percent protected against a recurrence of major depression during the next ten years. And those who were highly spiritual and had gone through a major depression in the past, had a 90 percent protective benefit against a recurrence of depression. The findings reveal that suffering appears to build a spiritual core within that prepares us for the next time we face suffering.

Miller also shares in her book that a colleague, Dr. Brad Peter at Colombia, had used neuroimaging to evaluate the brains of 131 subjects, half with a family history of depression and the other half were at low risk. Twenty-eight percent of those with parents and grandparents who experienced depression were found to have relative **thinness** of their brain's right cerebral cortex. The region of thinning was in the region where we process emotional stimuli. This was felt to show that depression is associated with a narrowing of the perceptual field and a distortion of our sense of relationship with others and the larger world. For Dr. Miller, this raised the question if there is a biological pathway for depression, could there be a biological pathway for spirituality?

What followed was an fMRI study of the brain's regions of perception, orientation, and reflection—the occipital, parietal, and precuneus regions known to be associated with depression. The study revealed that participants for whom spirituality and religion were highly important had a healthier neural structure than did those where spirituality and religion scored medium, low, or was of no importance. The high-spiritual brains had broad regions of cortical **thickness**, as opposed to those with little or no spirituality and religious faith. Miller observed, "For spiritually aware people across faith traditions—and including those without a faith tradition—the brain appeared able to protect itself from the long-standing neurological structures of depression."

This finding stimulated further study with electroencephalography (EEG) focusing on the religion of cortical thickness. The EEG findings revealed subjects with a strong personal spirituality had a high-amplitude alpha rhythm (8-12 Hz), a wavelength that is found in the brain of meditating monks. Miller called those with a high-amplitude alpha rhythm "**the awakened brain**" and was able to conclude: "Depression and spirituality appeared to be two sides of the same coin, vastly different experiences that in fact share some significant pathology." She even wondered "if some types of depression might be a symptom of a person's craving for spirituality and a call for the spiritual self to awaken." She took one step farther and concluded, "Spirituality is a consciousness for which all our brains are wired, and that, long-term, the spiritually engaged brain is a healthier brain." And "Depression could be a knock at the door for the opportunity of an awakened brain" (Miller, 2021, p 149-154).

Beliefs Affect Our Choices

Importantly, whether our beliefs are factually based or not, the beliefs we hold affect our values, attitudes, choices, judgments, and behavior. Some parents have the belief they should trust God instead of using vaccines to prevent disease. All too often, their children bear the effect of their choice by acquiring a potentially life-threatening attack with the measles virus. Conversely, scientists who focus only on the material universe, can dismiss encounters with the spiritual dimension in their own life and that of others. Furthermore, beliefs shape our personal self-identity and worldview, affecting every area of our life.

Like Piggy in the cartoon *Pearls Before Swine* by Stephan Thomas Pastis, those who suffer abuse early in life may develop a firm belief that they will always experience abuse. They may project this belief onto co-workers, neighbors, governmental programs, faith communities, and the universe. Aware of the bad things that happen daily, they may reject those who say, "God is good, all the time." Interestingly, individuals holding these opposing beliefs can find evidence in scripture to "prove" their point—that God is a good God or a wrathful God.

Individuals who are addicted to tobacco, alcohol or drugs, often hold the belief they are not an addict even though experiencing broken relationships, divorce, loss of employment, and bankruptcy.

Fortunately, many awaken and take steps (with A.A.) to restore their lives. In retrospect, they realize their earlier belief they were not addicted was a deception, an illusion.

A growing number of people hold to the belief that our planet and every human being and creature on our planet are worthy of respect, love, and compassion. Animal lovers are known to risk their own lives to rescue animals in distress. Today, many give time and money to save nearly 50,000 animal, bird, and reptile species approaching imminent extinction. Others support efforts to mitigate the effects global warming will have on our planet.

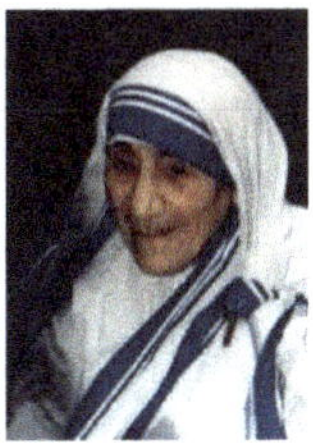

Mother Teresa Photograph taken at St Aloysius Church 19 I St NW, Washington, DC 20001 June 10, 1995. ©copyright by John Mathew Smith and given to the Public Domain, licensed under the Creative Commons Attribution-Share Alike 2.0 Generic license, Wikimedia Commons.

In 1946, Mother Theresa (1910-1997) had a profound experience that led to her serving countless homeless and dying individuals and orphans in Calcutta, India. Although she had taken vows of chastity, poverty, and obedience as a nun, she also professed her own fourth vow, "to provide wholehearted free service to the poorest of the poor." Over 4,000 nuns joined Mother Theresa in her work which continues to this day. She has been quoted as saying: "If we judge others, we will not have time to love them."

Personal Choices and Parallel Universes

Without a doubt, the choices we make change the direction of our lives and those we love. I will never forget when I was in the third year of high school my dad put three folding chairs in the front yard and had me, and my two brothers sit in them. It was a sobering moment when dad said, "Boys we haven't decided what we are going to do with you." I thought he was about to send us to reform school because we had been a handful to raise. But then he said, "We don't have a doctor in the family who wants to be the doctor?" I raised my hand and dad said, "Good, John will be the doctor." Next he said, "We don't have a dentist in the family, who wants to be a dentist." My brother David raised his hand and dad said, "Very good" and finally said, "We don't have anyone to carry on the real estate business, who wants to do that?" My brother Marshall raised his hand and that is the way things turned out. I became a physician, David a dentist, and Marshall entered the real estate world.

I have thought about this a lot. I loved the practice of medicine, but later in my life I felt God's calling to be an Episcopal priest. I wonder, what if my dad had said, "Who wants to be the priest in our family?" I am certain I would have raised my hand to be a priest. However, if I had gone to seminary early in life, I would not have attended Centenary College and would not have met my wife Pat. And I cannot imagine my life without my dear wife. And, if I hadn't married Pat our five children would never have been born. And I absolutely cannot imagine a world without Kirk, Cathey, Ginger, Margaret, and Patrick. So, choices matter, and in the context of this story, my father's choices affected all three of his son's lives from that moment on.

American theoretical physicist Michio Kaku, is among quantum scientists who believe that with every choice a **separate parallel universe** is created. According to this interpretation, every decision we make in life can create a new universe that splits off into a parallel universe. Each universe would then represent a different outcome from the other choices that could have been made. I believe scientists who hold this view may believe the choices we make in life are like entering another universe. The parallel universe concept is unproven and more philosophical than a scientific reality.

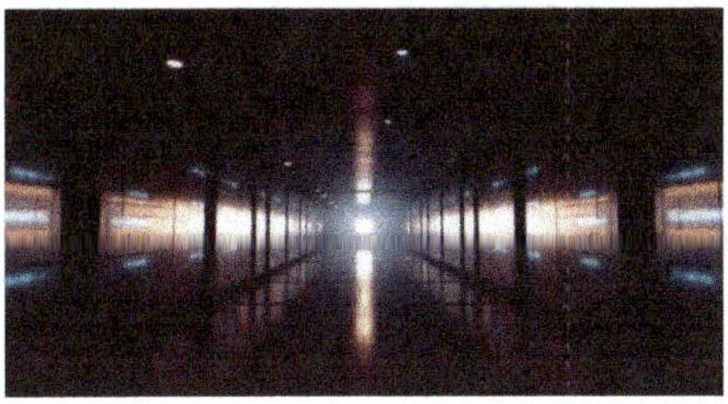 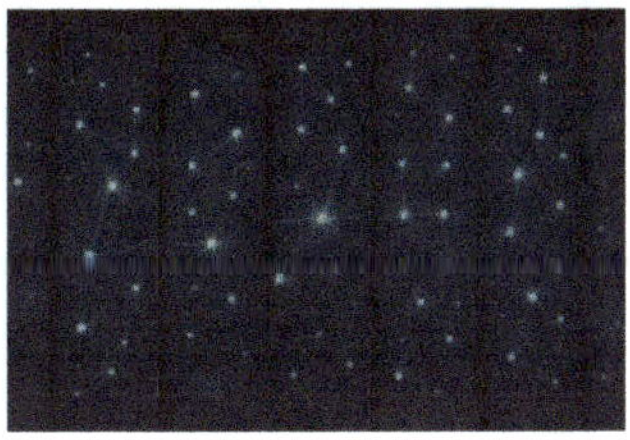

AI attempts to depict parallel universes taking place at the same time, but we are only in one.

Fiction writers have toyed with the idea of parallel universes in their books. Blake Crouch's book, *Dark Matter*, is the story of a man who had the choice of dedicating his entire life to being a research scientist and never being married but chose instead to marry the love of his life and has a son. He teaches physics in a high school where students could care less. Following an accident, he finds himself in a parallel universe—the sterile and empty life of the scientist he could have been. He fights desperately to return to his beloved home and family.

The consequences of the choices we have made have altered every aspect of our lives, and that can be pretty scary. Whether parallel universes exist, we are wise to consider the beliefs we hold and discern whether they are wise or not. But how do we do that? How do we challenge our own beliefs? I believe life has a way of bringing truth to us if our heart is open to receive the message as to whether our cherished beliefs are bearing good fruit.

Concluding Comments

Beliefs shape how we see the world—and how we see ourselves. Some are life-giving, guiding us toward love, truth, and healing. Others may limit us or be harmful to us and others. But all beliefs, even those that no longer serve us, carry the possibility of transformation. In the chapters ahead, we will explore where our beliefs come from, how they change, and how they can connect with the deepest mysteries of being. May we move forward with curiosity—and with compassion for ourselves and others.

If you'd like to explore your own beliefs more deeply, consider reflecting on the following questions. They are not meant to judge—but to illuminate.

- *Can you identify a belief you once held that no longer feels true? What changed? What led you to question it?*
- *Have others challenged your beliefs? Did that rejection hurt—or did it invite you to reevaluate what you hold to be true?*
- *Human beings are not perfect; we all make mistakes. Can you recall mistakes in the past that were a teaching moment for you? What beliefs were changed?*
- *Considering the impact of the choices we make, consider the choices you have made that changed the course of your life—the profession you chose, education you received, choice of a partner, and choice to participate in a particular religious community or not.*

Chapter 2—Sources of Belief

Where do our beliefs come from? Many will say, "I decide what to believe." Yet in truth, our beliefs are shaped over time by many voices outside ourselves—from our earliest moments that we are held in the arms of our mom and dad, to our everyday relationships and culture. As to having a "free will," Albert Einstein said, "Everybody acts not only under external compulsion but also in accordance with inner necessity." Einstein believed what we believe is determined by our nature or programmed into us from others. This is a disturbing thought, to be sure.

As social beings, we humans engage in a two-way and often emotional dialogue, which can strengthen and empower us to cope with the challenges we may face in life. Childhood experiences with siblings and peers, parents, and authority figures all play a key role in our initial understanding of the world and our place in it. Schools teach reading and writing, math and science, and we also are taught on the playground and in locker rooms the beliefs, attitudes, and behaviors that are acceptable within our own unique cultural setting.

As we mature, life continues to shape us. Education, relationships, and experiences—both joyful and painful—reshape our beliefs again and again. Our socio-economic context, the neighborhoods we live in, the friendships we choose and the co-workers we interact with each day have a profound influence over our beliefs and the choices we make. Furthermore, exposure to movies, books, art, crafts, the internet, and social media sites can either affirm or challenge our most cherished beliefs.

The Science of Belief

From the scientific point of view, beliefs are mental frameworks shaped by the complex interplay of neurological development (our brain is not fully formed until around age 25), environmental inputs, and social conditioning. Studies reveal that from early childhood attachment patterns to cultural narratives, from formal education to media consumption, the human brain continually assimilates, stores, and updates belief structures in response to experience. By examining the origins of our beliefs, we engage in a vital process that brings unconscious assumptions into conscious awareness. Our self-reflective capacity is critical for adaptive growth, moral reasoning, as well as emotional and spiritual intelligence. The more we understand the mechanisms behind belief formation, the better equipped we are to refine our perspectives in pursuit of truth, well-being, and a more inclusive human experience.

Porot and Mandelbaum (2019) observe that "beliefs seem to be a **critical nexus** around which the mind pivots." This powerful insight highlights belief as a central organizing force in human cognition. They further note that across fields—from comparative and computational psychology to neuropsychiatry, social psychology, and developmental psychology—belief cannot be excluded from the study of the mind; nor can belief be meaningfully excluded from everyday science.

Their research reveals that human beings maintain a "**web of beliefs**," a dynamic system where core beliefs are deeply integrated and defended, while peripheral beliefs are more loosely held and easily abandoned. This may explain a contradiction: how we can be quick to spot inconsistencies or weaknesses in the beliefs of others while ignoring the "web" of inconsistent or fragile beliefs that we hold ourselves.

Importantly, individual beliefs are not isolated; they are interconnected, influencing and reinforcing one another. When faced with a challenge to a particular belief, we often subconsciously draw upon what Porot and Mandelbaum call the "**wisdom of our belief crowd**"—the body of related beliefs and information we have accumulated over time to support our core beliefs. Interestingly, research shows that when individuals are asked to address the same question multiple times, their answers tend to progressively have greater clarity and accuracy. This suggests it is wise to pause for a moment before declaring a belief without consideration of its impact on others.

Together, these findings offer a powerful reminder: humility and kindness are not only virtues but are essential when our beliefs—or those of others—are questioned.

The Arts

Most would agree that the arts have been influential in our lives. Columbia College art historian, Rami Gabriel (2021) states:

> I argue that emotions evoked through ritual in art and religion play a significant role in belief fixation as part of the cultural evolution of imaginative culture. This is because participatory rituals compel feelings of immanence, which indicate heightened significance, or salience. This spiritual emotion composed of awe, wonder, and transcendence is the indwelling, inherent, the plenitude within.

I have always been fascinated by Michaelangelo, who psychologists believe suffered from clinical depression, yet he was able to spend four years laying on his back to paint remarkable frescos on the ceiling of the Sistine Chapel of the Vatican in Rome, and then another three years painting the wall over the chapel's altar. The frescoes depict the story in Genesis from Creation to the Great Flood. Michelangelo captures me when I view his depiction of the moment when God reaches out to touch the limp hand of humanity. The eyes of God and human are fixated on each other with expectancy, yet the two are separated by a gap that holds the mystery of creation. The painting invites me to imagine what is about to happen. Will God and humanity connect?

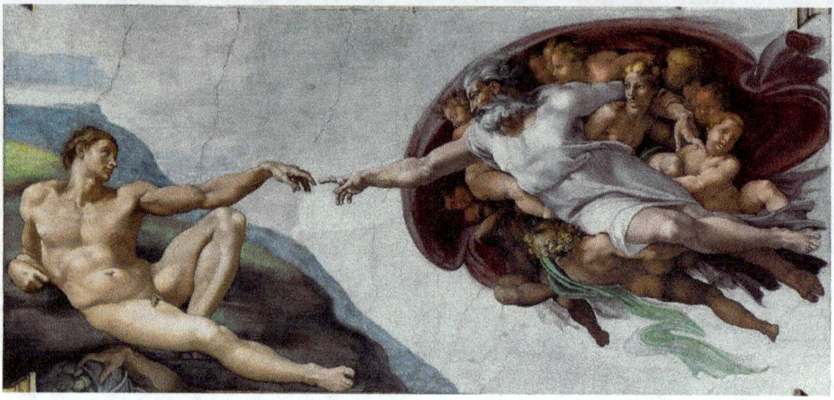

Michaelangelo, Sistine Chapel, God reaching out to Adam (1512).
Public domain, Wikimedia Commons

Religion and Beliefs

Equally significant is the formative power of participation in a religious community.

Pastwa-Wojciechowska et al. (2021) have written:

> For centuries, religion, piety, and spirituality have been the central point of human life closely linked to history and culture. In many cases, religion is the foundation of culture. It builds national identity and creates a sense of community.

The journey of faithful believers can provide a sense of connection to God and weekly religious services where there is corporate worship, singing hymns or chanting, prayer, reading passages of sacred scriptures, preaching, and a community of meaningful relationships. New attendees are often confirmed in a service and thereafter recognized as a fellow "believer." To believers in the church at Philippi, St. Paul wrote:

> Therefore, if you have any encouragement from being united with Christ, if any comfort from his love, if any common sharing in the Spirit, if any tenderness and compassion, then make my joy complete by being like-minded, having the same love, being one in spirit and of one mind. (Philippians 2:1-2)

Religious traditions can offer love, belonging, and moral clarity, but can also instill fear, guilt, or exclusion. Whether uplifting or burdensome, these spiritual influences often leave a deep imprint on our beliefs. When positive, they can nurture a loving life built on respect, empathy, and compassion. Unfortunately, that is not always the case.

Because most of us live our entire life in the same socio-economic and cultural setting, we may unconsciously or consciously develop prejudice and dismiss or reject those who are not of our persuasion. After all, the passage quoted above from Philippians encourages believers to be of "one spirit and one mind." This can easily lead to embracing an attitude that "our beliefs are the right beliefs." Beliefs that are inflexible, rigid and unaccepting of others are unhealthy and can be dangerous, leading to separation, conflict, and violence, even war. Furthermore, misinformation from authority figures, religious communities, and propaganda from media and political sources can shape and misshape our beliefs.

As mentioned in the previous chapter, beliefs affect every area of our lives including our values, attitudes, choices, and behavior. Our beliefs and the response of others to our beliefs can affect us mentally and emotionally. One thing is certain; we are responsible and accountable for our beliefs and the actions we take because of them. For this reason, exploring our beliefs is wise and allows us to continue to grow mentally, emotionally, and spiritually with respect, empathy and compassion for others.

Trust or Distrust in God

Rosmarin. et al. (2011) studied how the decision to trust or distrust God impacts spiritual and religious themes in the three main monotheistic traditions—Judaism, Christianity, and Islam. Trusting in God involves the belief that God is aware and taking care of one's interests; conversely, those who do not hold this view, assume God is either unaware or malevolent. The article mentions three core beliefs concerning the nature of the divine: (1) God is constantly aware and has regard for what is taking place on planet Earth; (2) God is omnipotent and in control; and (3) God is a merciful, loving God. Individuals who can affirm these core beliefs, not only trust God, but were found to have lower incidence of depression, anxiety and worry; conversely, those who embraced a distrust of God had higher levels of these symptoms. Furthermore, the authors state:

> A trust-in-God worldview in which God is seen to be fully knowledgeable, powerful and good may engender positive appraisals of events and thus decrease the need for certainty and predictability. Trust in God may also promote positive spiritual emotions, spiritual support, and a sense of connectedness with transcendence, thus increasing tolerance for uncertainty. Mistrust in God, on the other hand, may exacerbate intolerance of uncertainty by promoting fundamental questions, doubts, conflicts, and struggles with the Divine during stressful periods of life.

Personal Reflection

Perhaps no painting embodies more of the core beliefs of Christianity than that of The Last Supper by Leonardo Da Vinci (see next page).

First, Jesus is dominant, seated at the center of the table (Christ is central in the Christian story). Second, the painting depicts the story of Jesus' breaking bread and wine with his twelve apostles (bread and wine become the body and blood of Christ when received at Holy Eucharist / Communion). Third, the painting is about the great betrayal. Da Vinci has chosen to focus his painting on when Jesus has just declared that one of the twelve will betray him. The anxious reaction of the disciples is evident as they point and try to imagine who would betray Jesus. Finally, the betrayal (we learn is Judas) points to what will shortly happen though not depicted in the painting—Jesus' arrest and sacrificial death on the Cross—God's plan for the redemption of all people.

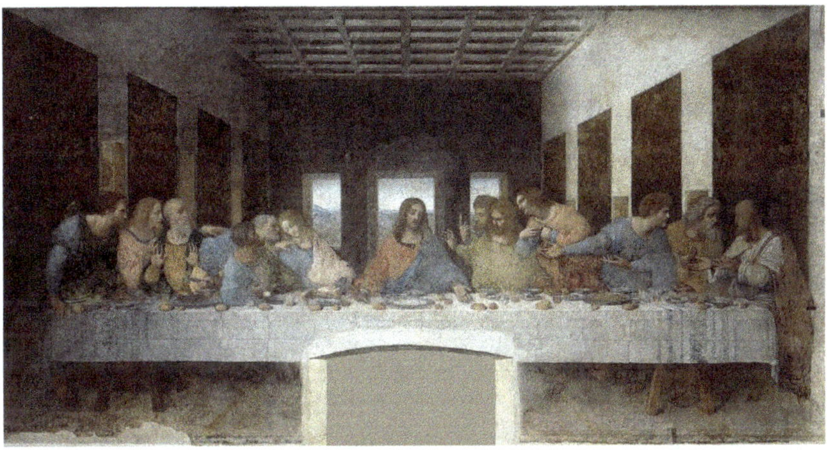

The Last Supper by Leonardo da Vinci – Mural inside the Dominican Convent of Santa Maria Delle Grazie, Milan, Italy.
Public Domain protected, printed unchanged. Wikimedia Commons.

Concluding Comments

Beliefs are much like a river, shaped by the lands they pass through—winding, deepening, sometimes diverted by storm or drought. They carry the sediment of our earliest stories, our kin, our fears, our hopes. The river is not fixed; it flows. As we walk its banks with curiosity, we may find some waters are clearer, others more mysterious. To trace the source of what we believe is not to dismiss it, but to honor the journey—to allow new springs to emerge, and stagnant pools to be renewed. In this sacred act of reflection, we find not just understanding, but the grace of becoming. The **journey of belief** is not a destination—it's a lifelong unfolding. As we reflect on the voices that have shaped us, we may find ourselves more open, more compassionate, and more curious. And that, too, is a form of grace. In the next chapter we will look at the transformative power of belief.

You may find it meaningful to pause and reflect on some of the following questions, not as a test, but to gently uncover the roots of what you hold most dear.

- *Porot and Mandelbaum talk about our "core beliefs" and the "wisdom of our belief crowd." Does this speak to you? If so, in what way?*
- *Can you recall a time in your childhood where an authority figure affirmed you personally? How did that make you feel? Did being affirmed have a positive effect on your self-esteem?*
- *Have you had a relative or friend reject a belief you hold as dear? What was that like for you emotionally and how did you deal with it? Have you been able to remain friends?*
- *In what setting are your beliefs affirmed and where are they likely to be rejected? Has that experience caused you to be attracted to some settings and to withdraw from others? Explore why some settings have attracted you and others have not.*

Chapter 3—The Physiology of Belief

What psychological and physiological mechanisms give beliefs their profound power in our lives? This is a compelling question, answered in part by "the placebo effect" in medicine.

During World War II, Dr. Henry Beecher, facing a shortage of morphine for wounded soldiers, injected some with a saline solution instead—telling them it was morphine. To Beecher's surprise nearly half reported relief of their pain. Today we understand this as the placebo effect: a demonstration of the power of mental belief to impact bodily function. Had Beecher told the soldiers that he was giving them salt water, the results would have been very different.

Power of the Placebo Effect

A dramatic incidence of the effect of belief on healing is the story of healing shared by Andrew Newberg, M.D., in his book Why We Believe What We Believe (2006). When first seen by an oncologist, every organ in Mr. Wright's body was riddled with metastatic cancer, and his physician said there is a new drug for cancer treatment called **Krebiozen**. After receiving injections with the drug, Mr. Wright's tumors shrank, and all signs of the disease disappeared. Two months later, the Food and Drug Administration announced that Krebiozen was ineffective. Hearing this, Mr. Wright immediately became ill with reoccurrence of his cancer. His doctor decided to lie and told Mr. Wright he needed to double the dose of Krebiozen and then it would be twice as potent. After receiving this double-dose, Mr. Wright went into remission for the second time with no sign of cancer. Later, Mr. Wright read an article in the newspaper that another cancer specialist said Krebiozen was worthless. Immediately, Mr. Wright became ill and died two days later. In retrospect, when Mr. Wright believed he was receiving a drug that would cure his cancer, his tumors when into remission and when he heard it was worthless, the cancer returned. Though a hoax, Krebiozen is a classic example of the Placebo effect (Benson, 1996).

A Harvard Medical School article entitled "The Power of the Placebo Effect" (2024), reviewed by Dr. Howard LeWine, affirms that our mind can indeed act as a powerful healing tool—even when the treatment is inert. While the article refers to placebos as being "fake treatments," I believe the real focus is to recognize the human capacity to heal through belief.

Physician, Eben Alexander, III, (2012) states:

> These studies open the door widely to the placebo effect, to the power of mind over matter, which modern medicine has acknowledged for decades in placebo-controlled trials. However, what most people fail to realize is that there are some extraordinary stories about the placebo effect where people completely cure their own cancer, infections, even some congenital deformities, and degenerative diseases.

The Science

In randomized double-blind studies, the power of belief—the placebo effect—in healing becomes evident. Participants are divided into two groups—one receiving real medication and the other, a sugar or bread pill. Crucially, neither the patients nor the doctor or staff know who is getting what. This is to ensure that every patient believes they are receiving the treatment in question. Routinely in such studies, 35–40% of those receiving only the sugar pill report healing or improved symptoms. And participants receiving the actual medication generally have only a bit larger number reporting improvement. The healing power of belief is obvious—both groups report improvement!

Understanding the power of the placebo effect, doctors and nurses are taught to remain calm, positive, and reassuring in caring for patients—even those terminally ill—because emotional tone can influence outcomes. A visit from a chaplain, a friend, or a faith community member, as well as their prayer, can activate this innate internal healing capacity all humans possess.

I once asked my son-in-law, a urologist, how he speaks to patients diagnosed with prostate cancer. He said, "I tell them that most of my cancer patients die of something else—and that they should go on and live a happy life." He watches as his patient's shoulders relax, and they smile. That shift—that breath of relief—is belief in action. The body's ability to heal has begun.

Our Body Heals Itself

When we accidentally cut ourselves, the wound will heal in a few days, with or without stitches. We have witnessed healing taking place many times but seldom consider our body's amazing ability to heal. On a larger scale, our immune system constantly rids the body of toxins, bacteria and viruses, and cancer cells are recognized and destroyed before they can multiply.

Belief systems influence us far beyond the psychological realm. They shape behavior, perception, and biological function. David Leong, Ph.D., of the University of Canberra, integrates neuroscience, neuroplasticity, and cognitive psychology in his work. He emphasizes the role of higher consciousness—an expanded state of awareness that transcends conditioned patterns and enables people to transform limiting perceptions into empowering beliefs. This transformation fosters growth and resilience both personally and professionally.

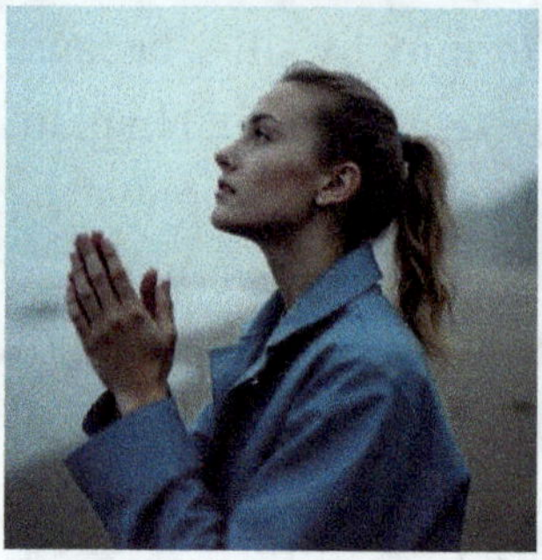

Woman Praying with Belief

Cell biologist Bruce Lipton (2016) agrees with this theme in *The Biology of Belief*. He reminds us that our bodies consist of roughly 50 trillion cells, each cell operating in a responsive, interconnected system. **Our beliefs**—both conscious and unconscious—interact with cells in every organ system of our body, influencing our biochemistry. **Neuroplasticity** allows new beliefs to rewire neural circuits, while limiting beliefs can instill harmful patterns that impede mental and physical healing.

Trauma and Homeostasis

Trauma, particularly when relational, can severely disrupt belief systems. Research shows interpersonal trauma—such as abuse, betrayal, or divorce—has deeper psychological impact than random accidents. Interpersonal trauma can devastate self-worth, distort perception, and alter one's core beliefs about self and others. These effects are often long-lasting and can shape one's health and relationships for a lifetime (Lopez-Martinez. et al., 2018).

Healing from trauma often involves restoring internal balance—what physiologists call *homeostasis*. The body continually regulates itself through a complex interplay of five major systems: the heart, lungs, autonomic nervous system (sympathetic and parasympathetic nervous systems), baroreceptors (blood pressure), and key regions of the brain. In addition, hormones like cortisol and adrenaline are released when stress activates the sympathetic nervous system's "fight or flight" response, while the "rest and digest" parasympathetic nervous system response with the release of endorphins, restores calm and supports the immune system. In chapter 12, we will review practices that can activate the parasympathetic response to retore one's homeostasis.

As Modell. et al. (2015) wrote: "Homeostasis mechanisms originated to keep a regulated variable in the internal environment within a range of values compatible with life." Organ coordination and cooperation sustains homeostasis day and night—largely without our awareness.

Biofeedback: Training the Mind-Body Connection

Biofeedback is a technique that trains individuals to consciously influence certain bodily functions—functions previously thought to only be automatic (Moss, 1998). Seen in this light, biofeedback is not therapy in the traditional sense of the word. Rather, much like going to the gym to strengthen our muscles, biofeedback offers a way to "train" physiological processes in our body to improve health and well-being

While typically not intended to replace conventional medicine, biofeedback has proven to be a valuable complementary practice. Research has shown that it can assist in managing a variety of physical, emotional, and mental health conditions, including high blood pressure, chronic pain, migraine headaches, anxiety, and stress-related disorders, with varying degrees of success (Frank. et al., 2010).

There are several different types of biofeedback, each focusing on specific physiological systems:

- **Thermal biofeedback** monitors skin temperature and has been helpful in reducing stress and anxiety.

- **Electromyography (EMG)** measures muscle tension and is often used to treat tension headaches and chronic pain.
- **Neurofeedback (EEG)** monitors brain wave activity and is applied to support insomnia, anxiety, and cognitive performance enhancement.
- **Respiratory biofeedback** helps regulate breathing patterns in cerebral palsy and stroke and is often used in anxiety reduction.
- **Heart Rate Variability (HRV) Biofeedback,** with many applications including cardiovascular, mental health, chronic pain, and prolonged grief.

Heart Rate Variability Biofeedback: A Window into Resilience

Heart rate variability (HRV) is not the same as the heart rate or pulse we feel at our wrist or monitor with a smartwatch. HRV specifically measures the tiny variations in time between each heartbeat—an essential marker of the body's adaptability and resilience. Surprisingly, a perfectly steady heartbeat is not the hallmark of health. Greater variability—small fluctuations between beats—is a sign of a cardiovascular system that is responsive to the varying energy demands placed on the body throughout the day. A reduced HRV has been associated with higher risk of morbidity and mortality, especially after events like myocardial infarction (heart attack). In such cases, a steady, inflexible heartbeat may predict poorer outcomes.

Thus, heart rate variability offers a crucial window into our autonomic nervous system's ability to respond to the changing demands of life.

Training for Coherence

Located in Boulder Creek, California, the HeartMath Institute is a nonprofit organization that has conducted extensive research since 1991 in HRV biofeedback. HeartMath has also developed accessible methods for training to achieve **The Coherent State**—a harmonious synchronization of heart rhythms, respiration, and blood pressure. When coherent, a sine wave pattern is seen.

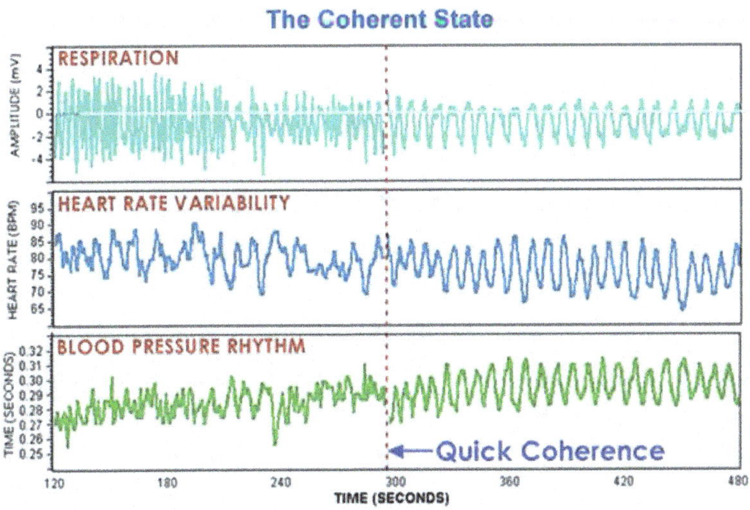

HeartMath.com, The Coherence State (May 15, 2025)

The HeartMath approach is non-invasive and cost-effective, making it well-suited for both clinical settings and individual home practice. Training typically involves:

- A small sensor is placed on the earlobe or fingertip.
- Software that provides real-time feedback on HRV patterns.
- Breath pacing to help individuals identify and sustain their "resonant frequency"—the breathing rate at which their physiological systems align most optimally.

During a session, participants are invited to:

- Focus attention gently on their heart center.
- Breathe slowly and rhythmically, imagining the breath flowing in and out through the heart region.
- Recall and evoke both negative and positive emotional memories, noticing how emotions impact their heart rhythm patterns.

As training progresses, participants learn to shift intentionally from **chaotic, erratic rhythms** toward a **coherent, sine-wave-like pattern**—an indicator of optimal physiological balance. The software provides visual feedback, allowing individuals to witness their growing capacity to regulate their emotional and physiological responses.

Through daily practice, many participants report greater emotional resilience, improved stress management, and a restored sense of agency over their inner experience. In essence, HRV biofeedback offers a doorway into the profound mind-body connection that ancient spiritual traditions have long taught—and modern science is now beginning to recognize.

Biofeedback offers an example of the transformative power of belief. It shows that when we become aware of our inner states, and consciously engage them with intention, we can alter our physiology, emotions, and even the experience of life itself. Whether through ancient spiritual practices or modern scientific tools, the message is the same: we are not passive recipients of fate, but active participants in the unfolding miracle of our own healing and growth.

Concluding Comments

Belief is not merely a thought we hold; it is a living force that shapes the body, stirs the heart, and guides the spirit. Neuroscience, psychology, and quantum biology all reveal that belief weaves itself into our very cells—molding new neural pathways, regulating emotions, and influencing the rhythms of our heart and immune system. Consider these points in your life:

- *We looked at the healing of a cut to recognize our body is "designed to heal." What do you think about how your body heals itself?*
- *Have you experienced the "placebo effect" in your life or that of a loved one?*
- *Why is it important to hear positive words from your physician? From friends?*
- *Biofeedback can awaken new patterns of healing and resilience. Have you experienced biofeedback*? If so, what was that like for you?

Final Word: Where our belief and biology meet, we find a profound truth: that with intention, hope, and love, we can help shape unfolding miracle of our own lives. May this understanding serve to welcome us to the next chapter where we will look at the transformative power of belief.

Chapter 4—The Transformative Power of Belief

Belief can be transformative. In his book *The Power of Art* (2006), Columbia University professor of art history, Simon Schama, describes great masterpieces as often anything but polite. He writes that the finest works "grab you in a headlock, rough up your composure, and then rearrange your sense of reality." Many of us have experienced this when encountering the artwork of van Gogh, Caravaggio, Rembrandt, or Picasso—a visceral feeling that the painting has captured our heart, mind, and spirit, and will not let go.

But where does the power of art come from? Schama answers:

> The power of art is the power of unsettling surprise. Even when it seems imitative, art does not so much duplicate the familiarity of the seen world as replace it with a reality all its own. Its mission, beyond the delivery of beauty, is the disruption of the banal... it throws a switch and generates an alternative kind of vision, a dramatized kind of seeing... van Gogh's paintings seem to exist in some parallel universe. It's as though our sensory equipment has been reset.

For me, Edvard Munch's painting, *The Scream*, has always had this effect. It pierces the soul, offering not just an emotional release but a mirror through which to understand suffering in a new light. Similarly, encountering the beliefs of others can "reset" something within us. It's as though we're offered new eyes, a parallel view of reality that challenges and expands our own. Belief, when it transforms, rewires our brain as to how we see, feel, and respond to the world.

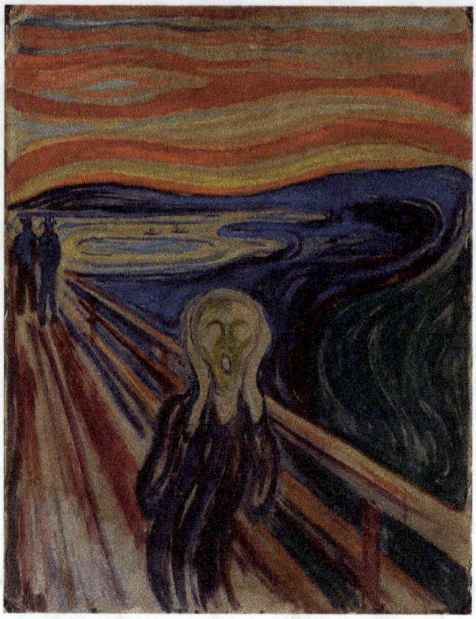

Edvard Munch (1863-1944), The Scream (1910),
Public Domain, Wikimedia commons. www.munchmuseet.no/en

Belief is Not Magic, Yet . . .

While powerful, belief is not a magic wand that can control all outcomes. Illness, loss, and misfortune still find their way into everyone's life. Yet, belief undeniably can shape our behavior, outlook, and resilience. Believing in oneself often leads to greater motivation and perseverance. Conversely, limiting beliefs can put a hold on one's progress and potential. When we encounter new ideas that challenge our existing beliefs, we experience cognitive dissonance—a mental discomfort that invites us to either adapt or retreat into rationalization. And beliefs, especially about ourselves and others, also shape our emotions. Believing we are loved fosters strength; believing we are forgotten can fill us with despair.

Transformative Power of Grief

Consider the experience of grief. Following the loss of a loved one, a widow may find herself not only facing sorrow, but the disorienting behavior of others. Distant relatives may arrive not to comfort, but to claim heirlooms and inheritance. Friends and neighbors vanish in silence, unsure of what to say or how to act. The bereaved is left in emotional exile. Stroebe. et al. (2007) report that "bereaved individuals have higher rates of disability, medication use, and hospitalization than the non-bereaved." The pain of interpersonal loss adds to the weight of personal grief.

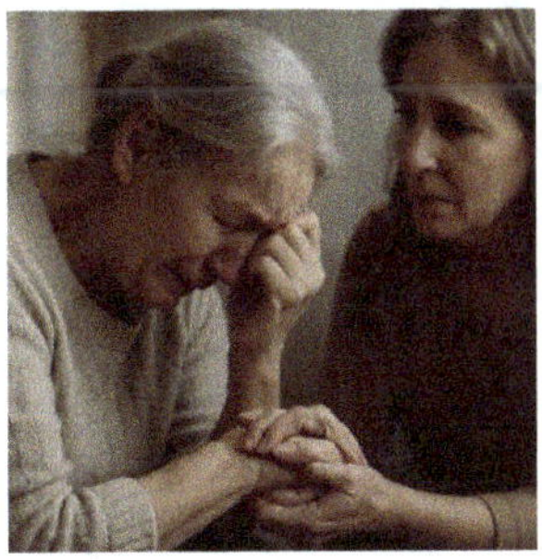

Woman comforted in her grief.

Yet positive transformation is possible.

After her husband's death, Theresa felt the sting of silence from friends who no longer called. But in that pain, she remembered times when she had gone silent in the face of another's grief. Theresa resolved to be different—to be present, to reach out, even when words failed her. "Now," she says, "I understand it's not about saying the right thing. It's about being there." In the power of presence, she discovered a new belief about love, one that reshaped her relationships and brought unexpected gratitude in return.

The Heart's Role

For centuries, across cultures, we've instinctively placed our hands over our hearts during emotional moments. We have all heard, "Out of the heart are the issues of life." But in the modern era, attention turned to the brain—to Freud, psychology, and the rise of cognitive behavioral therapy (CBT), mindfulness, and mental resilience. Only recently have scientists returned to the heart—not just as a pump, but as a center of feeling, memory, and wisdom.

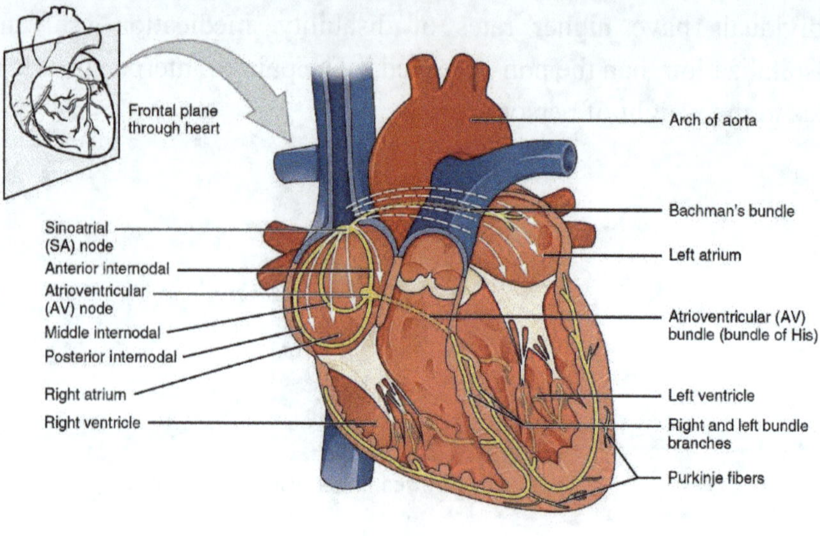

The Heart Neuro-Conductive System, Public domain. Wikimedia Commons. OpenStax College, Connexions Web site. http://cnx.org/content/col11496/1.6/, Jun 19, 2013. Licensed under the Creative Commons Attribution 3.0 Unrenewed license.

Discovery of the Intrinsic Cardiac Nervous System (ICNS) has sparked new interest in the heart's role in emotion, belief, and behavior. Cardiologist Giuseppe Giannino and his colleagues at the University of Turin (2024) describe the ICNS as a "**multi-level powerhouse**" that receives and integrates signals from both within and beyond the heart, generating autonomic responses that influence all cardiac function. Surprisingly, they observe that the heart exhibits both plasticity and memory—traits once thought to belong solely to the brain.

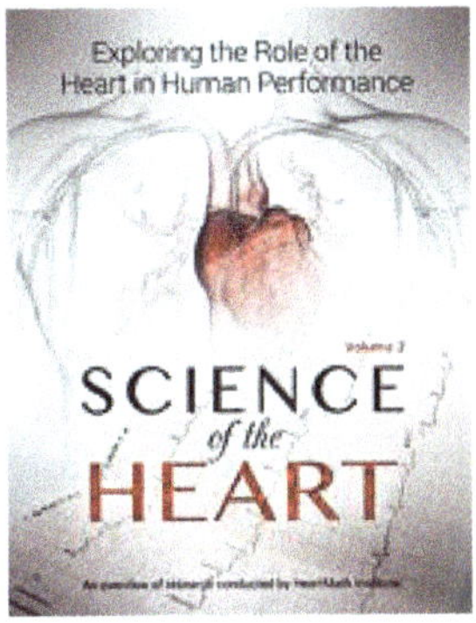

HeartMath.com

The HeartMath Institute in Boulder Creek, California, has spent over three decades researching the heart's role in human health and consciousness. According to their work:

> The human heart is much more than an efficient pump that sustains life. Our research suggests the heart is an access point to a source of **wisdom and intelligence** that we can call upon to live with more balance, creativity, and enhanced intuitive capacity. (HeartMath Institute, 2025)

Rollin McCarty, Ph.D., Director of Research at HeartMath, writes in his monograph *Heart-Brain Neurodynamics: The Making of Emotions* (2015) that the heart sends signals to the brain that influence cortical activity. When individuals focus attention on the heart while generating a positive emotion, it appears to *modulate brain processing itself.* In other words, emotions are not just born in the brain—they are shaped, and perhaps even guided, by the intelligence of the heart. This is more than metaphor. It is measurable. And it suggests that when you and I move our attention from our head to our heart, we shift the very landscape of our awareness.

Religious Transformation

Judeo-Christian: The Bible has many stories of transformation after an encounter with God. In the Jewish scriptures we learn of transformation in the life of Abraham, Moses, David, Jonah, and Ezekiel. In the New Testament, Mary, mother of Jesus, Mary Magdalene, Thomas, Peter, and Paul—after at first doubting God's call, each found the strength and courage to follow God's plan for their lives. In Romans 12:2 we read: "Do not be conformed to this world but be transformed by the renewing of your mind." These are words of transformation.

Hinduism: The 19th century Indian mystic, Ramakrishna, investigated many religions including Christianity and Islam prior to committing to Hinduism. This led to his belief in the unity of all religions. He is known to have had profound spiritual experiences and was a significant figure in the resurgence of Hinduism. Among the saying of Ramakrishna are: "The winds of God's grace are always blowing, it is for us to raise our sails," and "If you must be mad, be sure it is not for the things of this world. Be mad with love for God."

Islam: The Qur'an proclaims that God's grace is a gift, and individuals are encouraged to respond by following God's teachings and to seek a life of righteousness. Pursuing righteousness leads to transformation as individuals choose to surrender to God's will for their lives. The invitation to surrender is expressed in the Qur'an 2:136: "Say: We believe in God and that which was revealed to us, and that which was revealed to Abraham, Ishmael, Isaac, Jacob, and the tribes, and that which Moses and Jesus received, and that which the prophets received from their Lord. We make no distinction between any of them, and to Him [Allah] we surrender."

The Negative Power of Trauma: When Belief Is Wounded

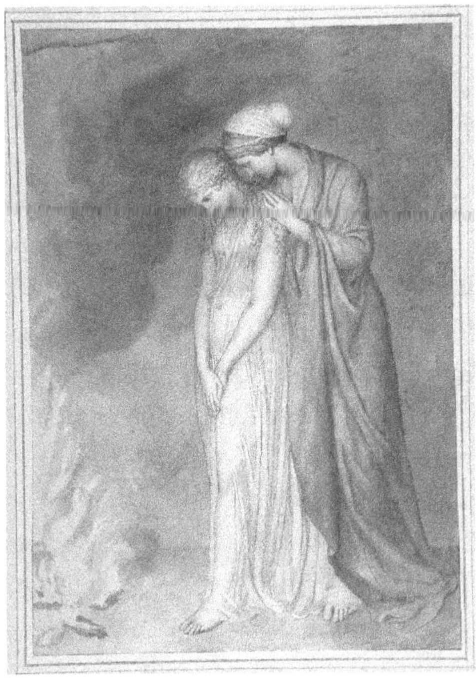

Study of Two Woman grieving, by John Flaxman Jr (1755-1826),
Public Doman, Wikimedia Commons.
Creative Commons CC0 1.0 Universal Public Domain Dedication.

As we celebrate the healing and transformative power of belief, it is also important to acknowledge the ways belief can be shaped—and sometimes wounded—by life's deepest sorrows. Beneath the surface of many broken dreams and life struggles lies a story of trauma, where belief, once a source of strength, has been twisted by pain. To fully understand the transformative potential of belief, we must also confront the darker reality: the way trauma imprints itself upon the mind, body, and spirit, shaping beliefs that can inhibit growth and suppress the soul's natural movement toward wholeness.

Traumatic events—particularly those that occur repeatedly or without resolution—can deeply shape the beliefs we hold about ourselves, others, and the world. Life experiences, both joyful and tragic, create thought patterns that are stored in memory, gradually forming the architecture of our self-identity. When negative experiences are repeated or left unhealed, the resulting beliefs become etched more deeply into memory, often reinforcing perceptions of fear, helplessness, or unworthiness.

Psychotherapist and trauma specialist O'Shea-Brown (2021) writes, "Complex trauma is insidious and pervasive in our society; it changes the way an individual perceives themself and others, in addition to adversely impacting how safe and secure one feels in navigating the world around them." Trauma can, therefore, act as a devastating architect of belief, building unconscious frameworks that sabotage our sense of safety, trust, and hope.

From a physiological standpoint, trauma triggers powerful survival mechanisms within the brain. In the face of overwhelming events, the amygdala—the midbrain's center for threat detection—is activated, while the hippocampus encodes these experiences into memory. However, traumatic memories often remain unresolved, buried in the unconscious mind, and lie dormant until later reactivation by seemingly unrelated triggers.

When trauma remains unresolved, it dysregulates the body's stress response. Upon encountering a new stressor, the body can enter a **hyperarousal survival state**—characterized by the "fight, flight, or freeze" response—through overactivation of the sympathetic nervous system (SNS). In healthy systems, the parasympathetic nervous system (PNS) provides a counterbalance, helping the body return to equilibrium. But in individuals with complex trauma, the PNS remains suppressed, unable to adequately soften or modulate the physiological storm. As a result, reactions to minor provocations may be intense, even violent.

This disconnection between stimulus and overwhelming response can bring profound confusion, guilt, and shame—not only to those suffering, but to their families and loved ones. Without healing, such cycles can lead to isolation, despair, and, tragically, suicide.

Recovery from the wounds of complex trauma demands more than mere intellectual understanding. It requires skillful, **multi-modal therapeutic interventions** that address both mind and body. Healing also asks for something deeper: profound patience, persistent love, and a compassionate and supportive community. Transformation is possible when individuals and families understand the roots of trauma, approach the healing journey with tenderness, and dare to believe in the capacity of the soul to be restored and made whole.

Concluding Comments

Belief is the hidden brush that paints the contours of our inner world. Like a great painting, it can seize us, shake us, and offer a new vision. Belief is the quiet architect of courage, the silent agent of fear, the compass by which we navigate joy and suffering. Now, science is catching up to what mystics, poets, and prophets have long intuited: belief is not merely a passive state of mind. It is a living force. It can rewire neurons, modulate heart rhythms, and awaken the body's healing potential.

Whether it is the heart's cry embedded in *The Scream*, the wise intelligence beating within our chest, or the still small voice of intuition—**belief transforms**. When nurtured with compassion, presence, and awareness, belief is no longer just a thought. It becomes a catalyst for healing. A doorway to wholeness. If you wish to explore further the transformative power of belief in your life, you may consider spending time with the following questions:

- *Can you recall a moment when a belief was transformative? What was that like for you? Did the transformation alter or affirm a core value you previously held?*
- *Have you or someone you know lost a loved one? What was the grief experience like? What are some ways to find relief? In this chapter Theresa gives some good advice.*
- *Heart-brain research reminds us that wisdom flows not only from the mind, but from the deep intelligence of the heart. How has your heart "spoken" to you?*
- *Have you or someone you loved experienced a traumatic event? What was that like and has there been resolution?*

Chapter 5—Beliefs Can Change

Even core beliefs are not set in stone. They evolve as we evolve. What once seemed true may no longer resonate. New insights, life experiences, and even pain can call our assumptions into question.

Neuroscientists Angel and Seitz (2024) describe belief formation as the human capacity to react to other brain functions such as perception, learning, memory, reward and loss computation, and deciding on choices for action. Much of this process takes place in the unconscious mind. We often discover—sometimes with surprise—that a belief we once held firmly has shifted.

The Global Mind and the Expanding Soul

Today, we are exposed to a global, interactive community through travel, the internet, media, and social networks confronting us with people who often think, live, and believe differently. Sometimes this broadens and enriches our understanding. Sometimes it is distressing. But inevitably, it changes us. And this change, like belief itself, can be for better or worse.

The ability to hear different voices from around the world has introduced humanity to a diversity of beliefs, customs, and rituals unknown in previous generations. The result is a global conversation that challenges our tribal notions and, at the same time, can awaken us to a deep longing for unity that exists in the heart of all humanity.

Beliefs can be strengthened through this exchange, refined into deeper wisdom. They can also be exposed as outdated or incomplete. At its best, this global awareness invites humility: What if I don't know everything? What if someone else's truth has something to teach me?

When Belief Transforms: Stories of Spiritual Awakening

Throughout history, spiritual leaders have experienced profound transformations in moments that shaped not only their lives but the course of cultures and civilizations (Kripal et al., 2024).

Siddhartha Gautama, the Buddha, was born into royalty and shielded from suffering. But when he ventured beyond the palace walls and saw sickness, aging, and death, something broke open inside him. He renounced his life of comfort and began a spiritual quest that culminated in enlightenment. The Buddha's teachings, Four Nobel Truths, Eightfold Path, and Five Precepts, born from his inner struggle, continue to offer millions a path toward freedom from suffering.

St. Augustine lived a life of pleasure and ambition, distancing himself from the Christian faith of his mother. But in a moment of deep despair, he heard a mysterious voice say, "Take up and read." Opening a Bible, he encountered a passage that pierced his heart. His conversion was immediate and life changing. Augustine became a foundational voice in Christian theology, a testament as to how even the most deeply ingrained beliefs can change under divine light.

Moses has a prominent place in all three monotheistic religions—Judaism, Christianity, and Islam. His transformation took place when God appeared to him in a burning bush and called him to lead the Children of Israel out of bondage. Moses resisted, but after God showed him miraculous signs, Moses led the Israelites through the Red Sea to the Promised Land. On Mt. Siani, he received the Ten Commandments from God and is found prominently mentioned in the first five books of the Bible as well as in the writing of the Hebrew prophets. In the New Testament, Moses and Elijah (representing the Law and the Prophets) appeared at Jesus' transfiguration on a mountain top (Matthew 17:1-5). Moses is mentioned more often than any other individual in the Qur'an where he is recognized as a prophet and messenger of God.

These stories are not meant to minimize the cost of change. In each case, the journey was marked by inner struggle, loss, and surrender. But they demonstrate what is possible when belief evolves in the direction of greater truth, compassion, and unity.

Changing Beliefs in Everyday Life

Belief change is not confined to the lives of saints or sages. It's something we all experience. Consider how society has shifted its collective beliefs in just a few decades:

- Mental health is no longer seen as weakness but recognized as essential to well-being.
- Racism and gender roles that once were widely accepted are being redefined.
- Climate change, once denied, has become globally a pressing moral and scientific concern.

These are not just social trends—they are massive, global shifts in belief. And they came through listening, protest, research, heartbreak, and courage.

On a personal level, you may find your beliefs have changed over time about politics, spirituality, science, or even your own worth and purpose. Perhaps a conversation, a crisis, or a book opened your eyes. Perhaps a loss opened something in you that could never go back to what it was. Below are two individuals steeped in science who changed their beliefs.

Dr. Michael Egnor, a neurosurgeon, was an atheist and did not believe humans have a spirit or soul. He now says that his everyday experience with neurosurgery patients; working with neuroscientists, doctors, and students; and through devoted study of two thousand years of philosophical discoveries about the human mind and soul, he has concluded that humans are spiritual beings created by God, destined for eternal life. His personal story is found in Chapter 13, Miracles Defined (Egnor & O'Leary, 2025).

Dr. Stephen C. Meyer changed his beliefs. In his youth, Meyer experienced anxiety as to whether he could find meaning or purpose in life. The books he read taught of an impersonal universe, devoid of God. However, in the Bible he found a personal God who created the universe and offered humanity eternal life after death. In a college philosophy class, Stephen realized belief in God had dissolved his fear of meaninglessness. After receiving his Ph.D. in the Philosophy of Science at Cambridge, Meyer now serves as Director of the Center for Science and Culture in Seattle, WA, and has written best-selling books to affirm the belief that the findings of science and belief in God are compatible. His latest book is *Return of the God Hypothesis: Three Scientific Discoveries that Reveal the Mind Behind the Universe* (Meyer S., 2021).

Chaos and the Science of Change

Briggs and Peat's (1999) book is entitled, *Seven Life Lessons of Chaos, Spiritual Wisdom From The Science of Change*. In the attempt to understand the causes of thunderstorms, turbulent rivers, tornadoes, hurricanes, and complex patterns from any cause, **chaos theory** refers to an "**underlying interconnectedness** that exists in apparently random events." Science looks for hidden patterns for how the unpredictable leads to new understanding. Here chaos is both death and birth, destruction and creation. In our body, cells are constantly dying and being replaced. And, psychologically, we are not the same person we were ten or twenty years ago. Cultures and relationships also change over time. New technologies create change and artificial intelligence (AI) will soon force radical adjustments for everyone. Will there be chaos? Probably, but scientific evidence indicates **chaos helps free us** from our status quo and invites us to envision reality as a flux of changing patterns enlivened by sudden turns. In other words, chaos shakes the very foundations of our certainty, demands humility, while creating new and creative ways of thinking. Instead of resisting chaos, we can choose to embrace it with a sense of expectancy.

Yet, certainty in belief is comforting; conversely, uncertainty can arouse a survival response. To challenge a belief—or to experience an inner shift—can feel as if we have entered chaos. It threatens the mental foundation we built over the years to make life manageable. The familiar, even when it no longer serves us, feels safer than the unknown.

Physiologically, resistance is wired into us. The brain's fear center, the amygdala, treats **uncertainty** as a threat to one's survival. Anxiety rises. We want to flee. Not because we are weak, but because we are human. In life we often face crossroads. Uncertainty. Which way?

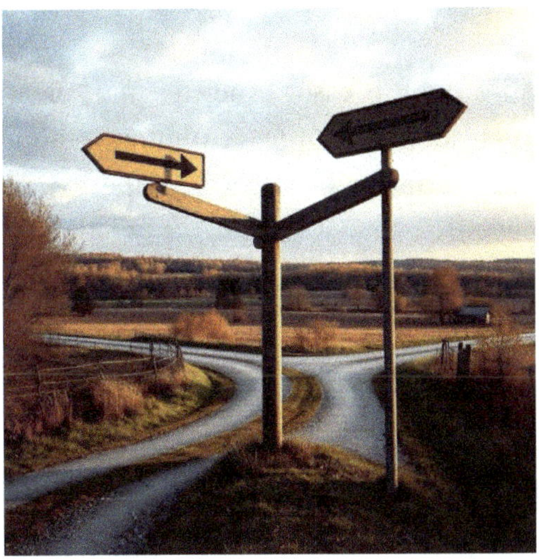

Life at the crossroads.

Porot & Mandelbaum (2020), state that the beliefs we hold dear are ones we associate with our **self-identity**—"I am a Christian!" A challenge to what it means to be a Christian can be perceived as a threat to one's very existence. Survival aroused! In much the same way as our ***body's immune system*** wards off attacks by bacteria, viruses, and toxins, when challenges occur to a core belief, our psychological immune system is activated to protect our beliefs from what is perceived as a major psychological threat. Our ***psychological immune system*** functions to help sustain not only our deeply held beliefs but also our very self-image.

Spiritually, this resistance can be seen as the individual's struggle between comfort and growth. The "former self" must, in a sense, die for the new self to emerge. Like any death, this transition is often painful and can be mysterious.

This is why transformational stories—religious and otherwise—are so dramatic. They often come at a breaking point, through crisis, loss, or an unexplainable encounter that overrides our defenses. When rigidity softens, change can enter.

Reaction to the Divine

University of California Professor Emeritus and scientist, **Dr. Valerie Hunt** (1916-2014) identified five common emotional responses people have when confronted with a genuine spiritual or mystical experience—especially one that challenges existing beliefs:

1. Fear – "My colleagues and friends will think I've become a religious freak."
2. Loss of control – "I don't know what God might ask of me."
3. Responsibility – "If I've received healing or insight, what now is expected of me?"
4. Disappointment – "God didn't answer me when I needed Him most."
5. Unworthiness – "God is great and wonderful, but I am weak and flawed."

These are real and valid responses. Encountering the sacred is not always comforting. It often destabilizes us—shakes our assumptions, reveals our lack of faith or trust, and forces us to reexamine what we really believe.

Reflection: Your Journey of Belief

Belief is not static—it is a lifelong unfolding for all of us—whether we realize it or not. As you reflect on your own journey of faith, consider the following:

- How have your beliefs changed over time concerning religion, race, sexuality, or other cultures?
- Can you recall a personal experience—a loss, a conversation, a dream—that reshaped what you believed?
- What does the picture below have to say about change?

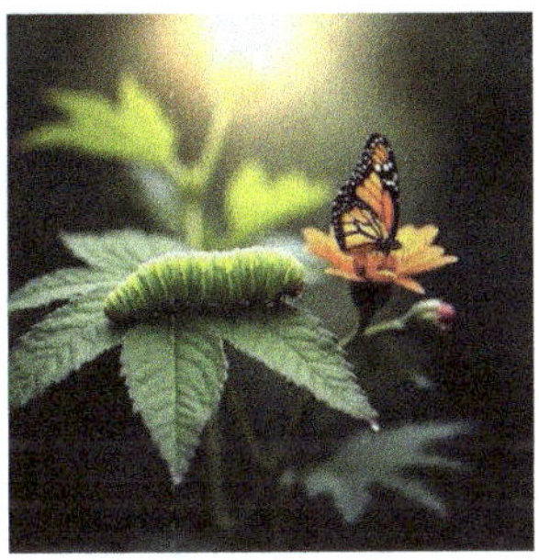

Caterpillar and butterfly

Concluding Comments

Even our core beliefs can and do change over time. Belief is not about having all the answers—it's about remaining open to the deeper questions that shape our becoming. Allowing mind, heart, and spirit to be open to new understanding is not only wise, but also an indication of spiritual maturity.

In the next chapter we will look at the impact of our personal beliefs. Before moving on, you may wish to ponder for a few moments and reflect on these questions which echo the content of this chapter and its message that beliefs can change.

- *Can you recall a major change in your belief concerning an issue? What was it like for you to realize you needed to change your long-held belief?*
- *Have you been exposed to someone from another culture who held beliefs that were different from yours? What did you learn from that experience?*
- *Spiritual leaders in major world religions have had an encounter with the divine that changed their beliefs and life thereafter—Buddha, Augustine, Moses, etc. What does it mean to you that individuals from very different backgrounds can have a transformative experience with their understanding of the divine?*
- *Dr. Valerie Hunt mentions five reactions that cause many people to back away from the divine—fear, loss of control, responsibility, disappointment, and feeling unworthy. Has this ever happened in your life, causing you to back away from giving yourself fully to God, your higher power? Does this concern still have the power to limit your relationship with God? If so, is it a valid response?*

Chapter 6—Personal Beliefs

We like to believe that we are rational, logical human beings, and that our beliefs are formed through careful consideration of facts. But, as mentioned previously, beliefs are shaped by lifelong experiences, emotional connections, cultural narratives, and social identities. When these beliefs are challenged, we tend to become defensive. Our minds search for arguments to support our position and poke holes in the opposing view. Instead of seeking truth, we often seek validation.

Is there a better way? Can we learn to hold our beliefs with both conviction and humility?

Scientific Beliefs Matter

To explore this, psychologist Gordon Pennycook and colleagues (2020) conducted a study with over 1,000 participants—half Democrats and half Republicans—on their moral, political, religious, scientific, and conspiracy theories. The survey posed difficult questions: Should abortion be legalized? Is global warming at least partly caused by human activity? Can vaccines cause autism? Should the death penalty be used to deter crime? Should same-sex marriage be legal? Is the Big Bang the best explanation for the origin of the universe?

Participants were also asked questions meant to assess their **openness to new evidence**: Should a person always consider new possibilities? Should people consider evidence that contradicts their beliefs? Is it important to persist in one's views even when faced with opposing data? These questions sought to measure the motivation and willingness to revise beliefs.

Surprisingly, Pennycook and his team found no single political or scientific issue that clearly separated Democrats and Republicans in terms of logical reasoning. While religious individuals tended to be more resistant to changing their beliefs, both political camps showed caution and conviction when it came to topics involving conspiracy theories, religion, or the paranormal. The key insight was this: People didn't just differ in **what** they believed, but also in **why** they believed. Participants who perceived themselves to be at the extremes of conservatism or liberalism tended to root their beliefs more strongly in their social identity groups and in the information sources they trusted. Importantly, the researchers concluded that beliefs form over time, influenced by personal history, community, and worldview.

The **point being**, if we had experienced a different personal history, community and worldview up to this point in our life, we would very likely have chosen to be participants in what is presently an opposing camp. That is a sobering reality that may be difficult to believe.

Political Beliefs Matter

One of the most profound examples of belief in action is found in the life of **Dr. Martin Luther King, Jr.** King's 1968 book, *Where Do We Go From Here: Chaos or Community?* was published posthumously and challenges the notion that the Civil Rights Act of 1964 solved racial inequality in America. King argued that legislative change was only the beginning; real equality required economic and social justice. He called on Americans—black and white—to believe in a shared future where poverty, discrimination, and injustice could be overcome by collective will. The choice, as he framed it is **chaos or community**. Dr. King's political beliefs were grounded in his moral and spiritual convictions. They drove him to risk everything for a vision of justice. King's life demonstrates that belief need not be passive—it can shape and change history.

Religious Beliefs Matter

In the previous chapter, we explored the lives of great religious figures like Buddha, Augustine, and Moses. Here, we turn to another transformative figure: **St. Paul**.

Born Saul of Tarsus, he was a devout Jew and a passionate opponent of the early Christian movement. As he later recounted in Philippians 3:4–7, Saul was "a Hebrew of Hebrews," a Pharisee, and a Roman citizen. Passionately committed to his beliefs, he believed the followers of Jesus were heretics and sought to stop the movement by imprisoning as many as he could.

But on the road to Damascus, Saul's path was interrupted. A blinding light knocked him to the ground, and he heard the voice of the risen Jesus asking, "Saul, why are you persecuting me?" Blinded by the bright light, Saul was led into Damascus, where a man named Ananias restored his sight and baptized him. Saul's name was changed. He became Paul, and his beliefs were radically transformed, as well.

Transformed, he now believed that Jesus was the Son of God, the fulfillment of divine promise. Paul became one of the greatest missionaries of the early Church, founding communities across the Roman Empire and authored many letters to the churches he founded. Paul's letters became the epistles in the New Testament. His story illustrates how belief can change in response to divine revelation, and how such a transformation can led to new meaning and purpose in life.

Spiritual Beliefs Matter

In the 5th century B.C.E., **Plato** identified **five transcendental desires**—the desire for perfect truth, perfect love, perfect goodness/justice, perfect beauty, and perfect being/home. St. Augustine and many contemporary philosophers agreed and have provided their own insight to affirm that these transcendental desires reveal that God is present in our consciousness, showing that we must be spiritual as well as physical beings. Fr. Robert Spitzer, S. J. (2023) says these human transcendental desires provide an insight into the nature of how God is present to us in our consciousness. If these desires are valid in our lives, then God for us is perfect knowledge, perfect love, perfect goodness/justice, perfect beauty, and perfect being/home.

Columbia University Professor of Psychology, Dr. Lisa Miller, gave a presentation to professionals at the Institute for Spirituality and Health (May 2, 2025) in which she said that her research found that with individuals who have had a sustained spiritual life for over eight years there is an 80% positive protective impact on psychological health and well-being. And "all the psychological scales indicate a sustained spiritual life carries a positive impact on the occurrence or recurrence of depression, and when the risk for depression is highest, a sustained spiritual life is even more protective for these individuals" (Miller, 2014).

In another article, Miller et al. (2019) write:

> Across cultures and throughout recorded history, human beings have reported self-transcendent spiritual experiences. Though varying widely in form, from ecstatic religious chanting to a felt oneness with the natural environment, these experiences share a perceived dissolution of the boundary between self and other and a sense of union with something larger than oneself.

Spiritual Struggles Happen

Ano & Pargament (2013) have addressed the predictors of spiritual struggles. Although statistics reveal the positive aspects of a sustained spiritual life, spiritual struggles are common. The source of origin is multi-focal including issues that are: religious, personal, social, and situational. Symptoms include confusion and doubt over religious beliefs and values, interpersonal relationships, sexual behavior issues, and thoughts about receiving punishment for perceived sins. Another factor is whether an individual has previously cultivated coping strategies or has a social support network prior to experiencing their spiritual struggle. Also, situational issues that are interpreted to be unjust, unfair or uncontrollable are common predictors of spiritual struggles.

Ano and Pargament (2013) have identified **thirteen predictors** of spiritual struggle: (1) negative God Image, (2) insecure religious attachment, (3) negative attitudes toward their religious community, (4) a weak family-of-origin religious history, (5) neuroticism, (6) pessimism, (7) trait anger, (8) lack of social support, (9) loneliness, (10) having a situation negatively impact one's life, (11) "shaking up" one's life, (12) unjust or unfair events, and (13) uncontrollable. The strongest predictor in the study was when an individual accepted a negative appraisal of a situation in their life.

As opposed to routine life issues, the unique aspect about spiritual struggles is they bring into question beliefs about the very **nature of God** who was believed to be an all-powerful and all-loving God that would have protected the individual from what has become a crisis of faith. Unresolved spiritual struggles can lead to depression, anxiety, lower self-esteem, and when prolonged, likely an increased incidence of morbidity and mortality, including suicide. Although spiritual struggles are unique, it is common for individuals to approach these issues the same way they previously were able to solve problems in their life. Yet, those coping skills are unlikely to provide a clear path out of spiritual struggles, leaving the individual with little hope of resolution.

So, what is to be done for individuals who experience spiritual struggles? Clearly, a major implication gained from the study is that it is important to assess which of the predictors are at work for a particular individual. Comprehensive treatment can then focus on the areas involved while enhancing religious, personal, and social resources that can be strengthened. In particular, it is wise to gently explore the individual's beliefs as to the nature of God, while assisting them to know they are not alone and that tragedy is part of the human condition.

In another article, Pargament et al. (1998), have discussed the management of spiritual struggles following the 1995 Oklahoma City Bombing. Timothy McVeigh's hatred of the federal government resulted in 168 deaths, including 19 children, and several hundred injuries.

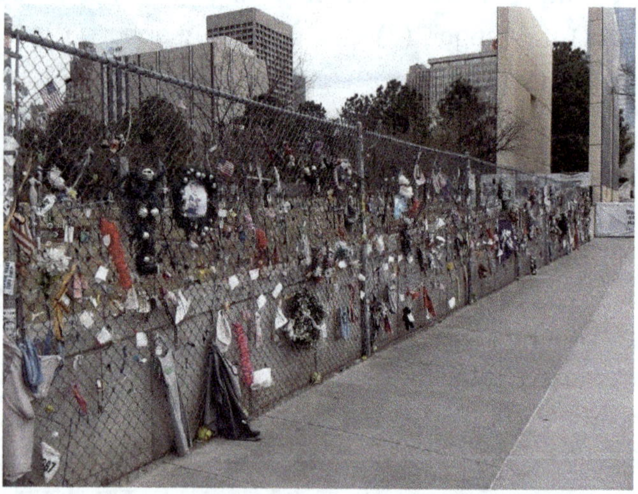

Oklahoma City Bombing Memorial Fence, 1995, Public Domain licensed under the Creative Commons Attribution-Share Alike 4.0 International license. Wikimedia Commons.

The findings and recommendations from their study provides guidance as to interventions that are warranted when someone is dealing with prolonged spiritual struggles. A **positive response** to the bombing was seen in those individuals who manifested religious forgiveness, sought spiritual support, participated in collaborative religious coping events, maintained their spiritual connection with God, prayed for religious purification, and had a loving religious reappraisal. A **negative pattern** was seen in those who experienced spiritual discontent, viewed the bombing a punishing God's act, interpersonal religious discontent, focused on demonic evil, and reappraisal of God's powers. Among the people interviewed, more individuals made use of the positive than the negative religious coping.

The study revealed whether individuals chose the positive or the negative coping pattern, had very different implications for their health and return to their pre-bombing life. In the same way, individuals who experience spiritual struggles and accept the positive pattern described above will typically have healthier outcomes—mentally, emotionally, and spiritually.

In the book of Genesis, Jacob wrestled with God's call on his life (Gen 32:22-31), and for many there is no greater struggle than to discern God's will and plan for our life.

Concluding Comments

With this chapter, we close Part I: The Power of Belief. We have examined belief from many angles—its origins, its physiology, its role in personal transformation. We've seen how beliefs shape nations and spiritual movements, how they are passionately defended, and how they can be transformed.

Now, as we move into Part II: Mystery, we step into realms that defy easy explanation. Mystery is not the absence of understanding, but an invitation to a deeper kind of knowing—one that welcomes awe, wonder, and the unknown. Let us now journey into the mysteries that surround us and see how belief opens the door to profound spiritual insight.

Before we journey into the next sections of this book—Mystery, Miracles, and Eternity—take this moment to pause and reflect on our own beliefs. Like the participants in Pennycook's study, we all hold core convictions. But how open are we to looking at them? Can we listen to differing perspectives with grace and curiosity? Are we willing to examine the sources of our beliefs and ask ourselves why we hold them so tightly?

Faith or strong confidence is a measure of the strength of our beliefs. See Hebrews 11 below.

Hebrews 11:1-16

1 Now faith is the substance of things hoped for, the evidence of things not seen.

2 For by it the elders obtained a good testimony.

3 By faith we understand that the worlds were framed by the word of God, so that the things which are seen were not made of things which are visible.

4 By faith Abel offered to God a more excellent sacrifice than Cain, through which he obtained witness that he was righteous, God testifying of his gifts; and through it he being dead still speaks.

5 By faith Enoch was taken away so that he did not see death, "and was not found, because God had taken him"; for before he was taken he had this testimony, that he pleased God.

6 But without faith it is impossible to please Him, for he who comes to God must believe that He is, and that He is a rewarder of those who diligently seek Him.

7 By faith Noah, being divinely warned of things not yet seen, moved with godly fear, prepared an ark for the saving of his household, by which he condemned the world and became heir of the righteousness which is according to faith.

8 By faith Abraham obeyed when he was called to go out to the place which he would receive as an inheritance. And he went out, not knowing where he was going.

9 By faith he dwelt in the land of promise as in a foreign country,
dwelling in tents with Isaac and Jacob, the heirs with him of the same
promise;
10 for he waited for the city which has foundations, whose builder
and maker is God.
11 By faith Sarah herself also received strength to conceive seed,
and she bore a child when she was past the age, because she judged
Him faithful who had promised.
12 Therefore from one man, and him as good as dead, were born as
many as the stars of the sky in multitude—innumerable as the sand by
the seashore.
13 These all died in faith, not having received the promises, but
having seen them afar off were assured of them, embraced them and
confessed that they were strangers and pilgrims on the earth.
14 For those who say such things declare plainly that they seek a
homeland.
15 And truly if they had called to mind that country from which they
had come out, they would have had opportunity to return.
16 But now they desire a better, that is, a heavenly country.
Therefore, God is not ashamed to be called their God, for He has
prepared a city for them.

As you ponder this passage, consider the following:

- *Do you agree that faith or confidence is a measure of strength of one's beliefs?*
- *Think about your core beliefs, and where do you think they came from?*
- *If beliefs shape attitudes, values, emotions, and behaviors, how might this insight influence your daily life or relationship?*

PART II: MYSTERY

Introduction to Part II, Mystery

In Part I, we explored the power of belief—its sources, its impact on our lives, and the transformation that can occur when our deepest beliefs shift. As we now turn toward Mystery, Miracles, and Eternity, an open mind and heart will serve us well. These subjects stretch far beyond what we can measure or prove. They require not only reason but imagination, wonder, and humility.

In Part II, we explore the concept of Mystery—those experiences, phenomena, and questions that defy explanation and dwell at the edges of our understanding. The human impulse to solve and define is strong—we create theories, systems, and explanations to banish the discomfort of not knowing. Yet despite all our intellectual tools, questions persist.

Quantum physicist Richard P. Feynman has said that for scientists:

> "Awe and mystery come again and again when we look at any problem deeply enough. With more knowledge comes deeper, more wonderful mystery, luring one on to penetrate deeper still. Never concerned that the answer may prove disappointing, but with pleasure and confidence we turn over each new stone to find unimagined strangeness leading to more wonderful questions and mysteries—certainly a grand adventure (Feynman, 1955).

In the chapters ahead, we will explore how mystery invites awe, wonder, and humility; how mystics and scientists alike seek to uncover the unseen; and how embracing mystery may bring us closer to truth than certainty ever could.

Chapter 7—Mystery Defined

Who hasn't looked at the deep-space images from the James Webb Space Telescope with a sense of awe and wonder? The swirling galaxies, the nebulae aglow with stars in formation—these photographs overwhelm the imagination. And now, physicists tell us that most of the universe consists of dark matter and dark energy, invisible even to our most powerful instruments. If ever there were a modern example of mystery, this is it. It's both unsettling and compelling—like a novel that refuses to give away its ending.

So, what is mystery? While definitions can vary across disciplines—scientific, philosophical, and religious—mystery, is at its core, that which eludes our grasp. It resists explanation. It provokes existential questions: Where did the universe come from? Does God exist? What happens when we die? Far from being irrelevant, these questions shape how we live. Mystery is not a gap in knowledge to be closed, but a threshold to deeper awareness.

Myths and Mysticism: Pathways into Mystery

Myths, when properly interpreted, should not be regarded as literal historical records. Instead, they serve as potent symbolic and metaphorical instruments that assist in understanding and navigating the complexities of human existence. They are vessels of cultural wisdom, expressing deep truths about the origins of the world, the nature of the divine, and the meaning of life. Through story and symbolism—whether in ancient epics or modern tales like *Harry Potter* and the *Life of Pi*—myths mirror the archetypal hero's journey: the struggle, transformation, and ultimate triumph over darkness.

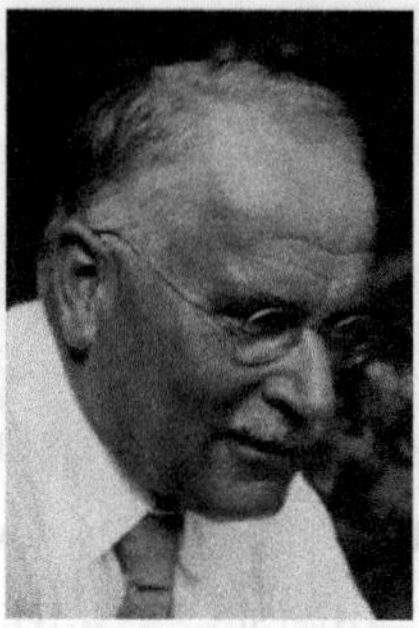

Carl G. Jung, 2010, Public domain, Wikimedia Commons

Psychologist Carl Jung believed that myths arise from the collective unconscious—a shared, inherited reservoir of archetypes and primal images that shape human thought and behavior. "We do **not invent** myths," Jung wrote, "we **experience** them" (Jung, 2009). They are expressions of something ancient and eternal moving within us.

Like myths, mysticism seeks to connect us with a deeper understanding of reality. It is one of humanity's oldest responses to mystery—an inner journey that bypasses rational analysis in favor of a direct and often amazing experience. Mystics endeavor to transcend the boundaries of the five senses and encounter a reality beyond dogma or doctrine. Through practices like prayer, meditation, contemplation, and visualization, mystics seek direct union with the divine—**ultimate truth**—with a form and means of communication that is deeper than words.

Mysticism is one of the oldest ways humans have explored the unknown. To repeat, mysticism wants to bypass intellectual analysis in favor of direct experience—seeking to know ultimate reality through spiritual practice, not rational thought. Mystics aim to transcend the five senses and access a truth deeper than words, beyond religious dogma or scientific theories.

In Christianity, mysticism takes the form of contemplative prayer and union with God. In Buddhism, it may involve the realization of emptiness and radical interconnectedness. In both, the goal is not knowledge in the conventional sense, but heightened awareness and the transformation of consciousness.

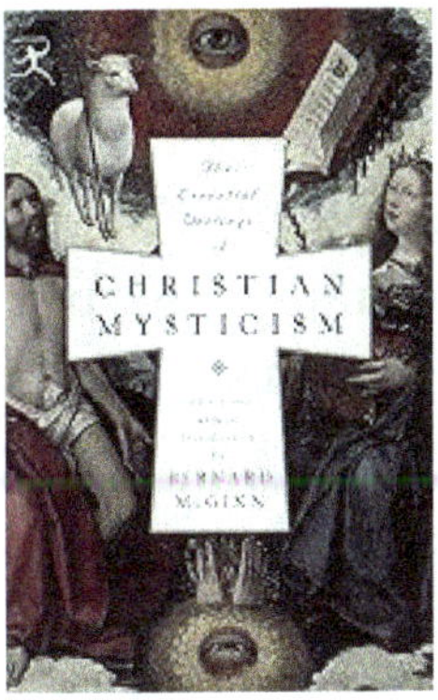

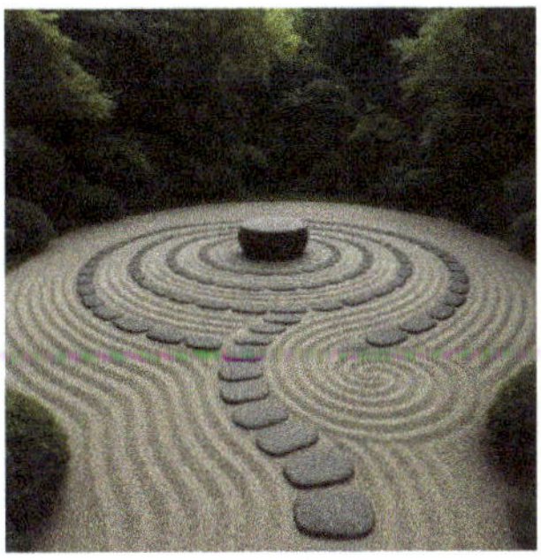

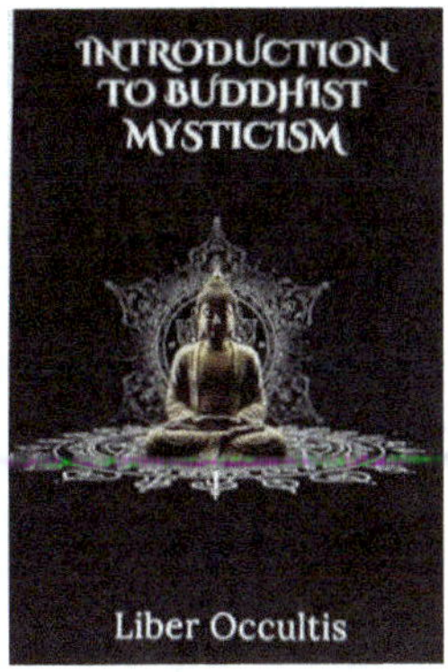

Interestingly, recent developments in quantum science—the informational universe, non-locality, and holography—echo ancient mystical insights. Many in the West are finding that modern physics affirms teachings found in texts like the *Bhagavad Gita* or the *Vedas*, often described as "the science of self-realization." The Bhagavad Gita presents a holistic approach to self-realization, encompassing knowledge, devotion, action, and meditation, all of which contribute to a deeper understanding of oneself and one's place in the universe.

Science: A Tool for Unraveling Mystery

Science, from the Latin *scientia* meaning "to know," is the structured pursuit of understanding. It offers powerful methods for solving problems—but it's also driven by the desire to illuminate the unknown. In this sense, science is a response to mystery.

For me, this yearning to explore life's mysteries is what led me to become a physician, an Episcopal priest, and later to serve as President of the Institute for Spirituality and Health at the Texas Medical Center in Houston. My life's work has been about serving those who face suffering—physical, emotional, and spiritual—and walking with them into life's deepest questions.

I recently watched an illuminating YouTube interview with Dr. Michael Levin, a brilliant biologist at Tufts University. His work on the mystery of **regeneration**—how salamanders regrow limbs and how planaria regrow brains—raises profound questions (Levin, 2022). He asks, "How does a salamander know when to stop regenerating?" "Why doesn't it keep growing more limbs and fingers?" Levin suggests the regeneration process is not directed centrally by the brain. Instead, he believes the process is directed by what he calls **cellular intelligence**—a mysterious, coordinated, collective awareness among cells that make up the salamander's arm. If understood, this process could someday lead to breakthroughs in human limb regeneration. Here again, mystery fuels scientific discovery.

Bridging Science and Spirituality

Most of today's mainstream scientists operate from a materialist worldview—one that focuses solely on the physical universe, often excluding the spiritual or mystical. But this is changing.

Gayle Kimball, a professor at California State University, has published dialogues with nineteen pioneering scientists who propose a new paradigm—one that integrates quantum physics, consciousness, and the spiritual dimensions of life (Kimball, 2021). These thinkers invite us to expand our understanding of reality beyond what materialism can offer.

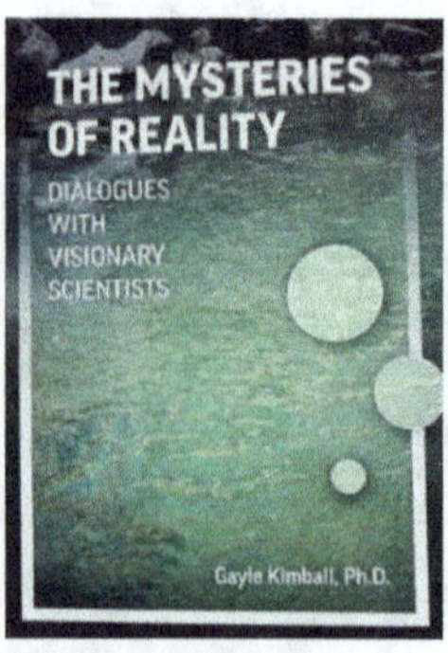

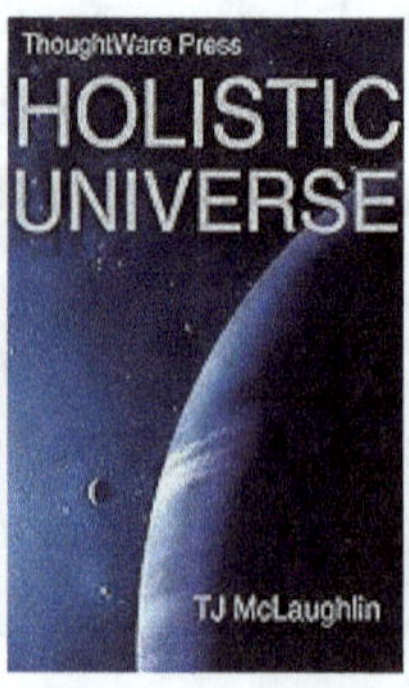

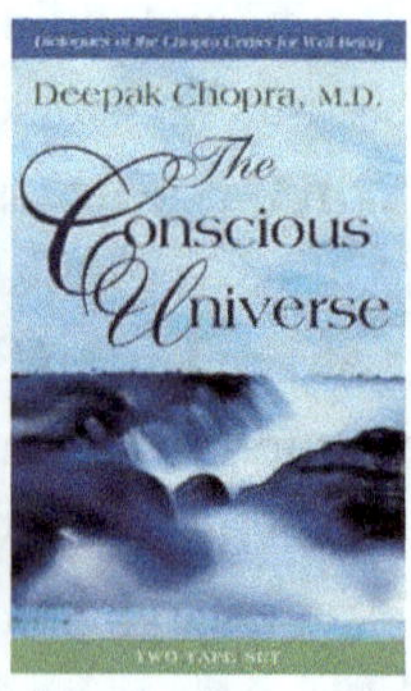

I resonate deeply with this **paradigm shift**. I affirm the physical universe—but I also believe there is a spiritual dimension equally real and vitally important to explore. This more holistic view—the union of material and spiritual realities, oneness and consciousness, in an Information Universe—will guide the rest of this book.

Dr. Dirk Meijer, Professor Emeritus in the Netherlands, is one such pioneer. He proposes that consciousness interfaces with a universal field of information (Meijer, 2012). Human awareness, in this view, arises from the way our brain reduces quantum possibilities into coherent experiences. In other words, we are not separate from the universe—we are embedded in its fabric, connected to its Ultimate Source, what some of us call God. From this perspective, the universe is **not random or meaningless**, but **informed, conscious, and evolving**.

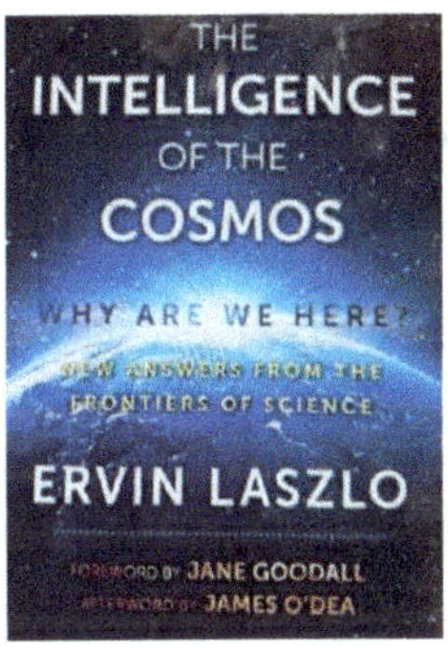

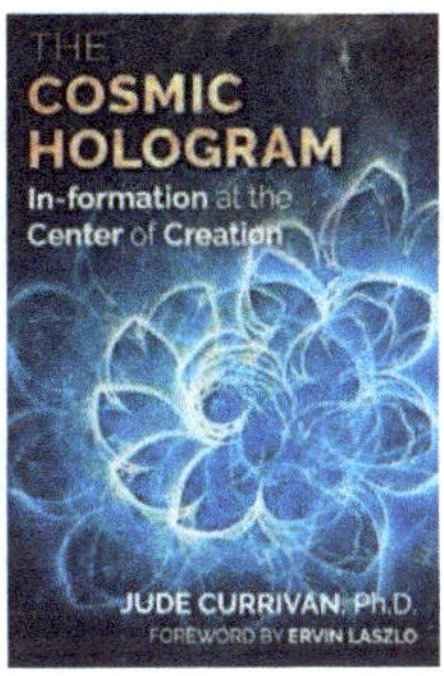

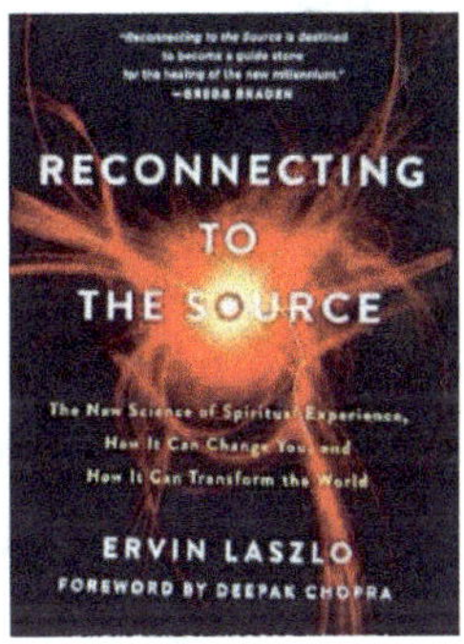

The Mystery of Our Own Lives

While we may be the most evolved species on Earth, many people are trapped and confined by cultural, political, or religious narratives. Some feel life is ruled by chance, or worse, by malevolent forces. But insights from neuroscience, quantum physics, and ancient wisdom suggest something radically **more hopeful**: we are **co-creators** of our experience.

Our thoughts, emotions, and moment-by-moment choices shape our reality. If true, this is an invitation to live with awareness and intentionality—to write a new script that is meaningful and life-giving, for us, those we love, and the world we share.

Concluding Comments

This has been just a glimpse of what is to come. The chapters ahead will explore these ideas more deeply. My hope is that you will find them both intellectually stimulating and spiritually affirming. The **emerging science offers a framework** in which the mystical, the miraculous, and the eternal are **not fantasies**—but **profound aspects of reality**, long explored by seers and sages, now coming into clearer view. Let us continue the journey—into the great mysteries of life.

Before moving on I have one question I hope you will consider thoughtfully. The question is:

- *Do you believe science and spirituality can unite? Think about it and you may want to reserve your final opinion until after you finish reading this book.*
- *Carl Jung said, "We do not invent myths, we experience them." What are your thoughts about experiencing myths?*
- *Is our universe random and meaningless, or informed, conscious, and evolving? What are your thoughts?*

Chapter 8—The Great Mysteries of Life

From the dawn of human history, we have gazed up at the stars, across oceans, and into our own hearts, compelled by questions for which we have no easy answers. Why are we here? What lies beyond this life? What existed before the beginning? These questions are more than intellectual curiosities; they are the deep stirrings of the soul—echoes of something greater that calls us to seek, search, and imagine. In this chapter, we will explore some of the most enduring mysteries that have shaped human inquiry across cultures and centuries. Though science has brought astonishing advancements, many of life's most profound questions remain unsolved. Perhaps they are meant to remain that way, nudging us toward humility, awe, and deeper reflection.

The Origin of the Universe

The Big Bang theory remains the most widely accepted explanation for the birth of the universe. But what caused the Big Bang? What existed before it? Did time itself have a beginning, or is it part of an even grander cosmic cycle we have yet to understand? Despite our powerful telescopes and precise measurements, the ultimate origin of the universe eludes us. Some scientists speculate about quantum fluctuations or multiverses, while others turn to universal consciousness and a divine, theological, or metaphysical explanation. Whatever the case, the sheer mystery of a universe emerging from apparent nothingness remains one of the most staggering enigmas we face (Swimme & Tucker, 2011).

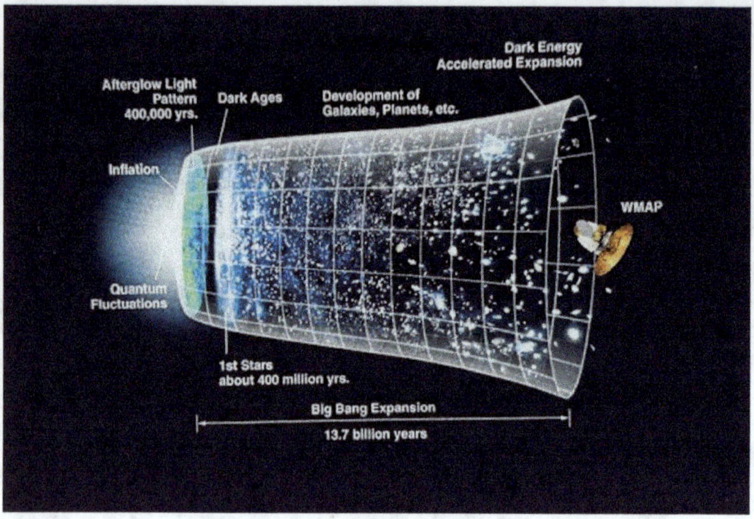

This graphic shows a timeline of the universe based on the Big Bang theory and inflation models.
(Image credit: NASA/WMAP)

What About the Six Days in Genesis?

Why does the first chapter in the Bible say there were only six days of creation, while science has found it took billions of years? First, many take Genesis literally and affirm it only took God six 24-hour days to create the universe. They say, after all, God can do anything. Second, some envision each of the six days as representing six eras where each "day" of creation represents millions or billions of years. Third, others have said Genesis can best be interpreted metaphorically to affirm that God's plan included us at the very inception of creation. Above all, Genesis speaks of God's love in creating the earth, its oceans, its land masses, its plants, its creatures and humankind. God created and said it was good. Hopefully, we can all agree creation was a good thing.

The Origin of Life

From lifeless matter to self-replicating, conscious beings—how did life arise on Earth? Was it a fortunate accident, the result of billions of years of chemical reactions in a primordial soup? Or was it seeded from elsewhere in the cosmos through panspermia? Some believe the findings of a dynamic and creative intelligence throughout the universe (DNA in cells and sub-atomic qubits) indicates a divine plan from the very moment of the Big Bang. Scientists continue to search for signs of life on Mars and distant planets, hoping to find clues that may shed light on our own beginnings. But the leap from non-living atoms and molecules to living cells is a chasm we have yet to bridge with certainty. The origin of life remains a sacred mystery, the most intimate of all.

Consciousness

Despite remarkable advances in neuroscience, the nature of consciousness remains elusive. How do electrical impulses in the brain give rise to thoughts, emotions, memories, and a sense of self? Is consciousness a byproduct of brain activity, or does it exist independently, perhaps as a fundamental feature of the universe as some quantum theorists propose? Mystics, philosophers, and scientists alike have wrestled with this mystery for centuries. Consciousness may be the one thing we experience most directly and yet understand the least.

This nature of consciousness mirrors the larger mysteries of our existence, which provoke questions that often transcend the boundaries of empirical science and venture into philosophy and spirituality. These inquiries—about purpose, origins, and the limits of what we can know—are deeply interwoven with our shared human experience. They invite us to contemplate not just the mechanics of the universe, but the profound implications of our place within it. As we navigate the uncertainties, we are beckoned not to merely solve these mysteries, but to embrace them as essential threads in the tapestry of existence.

The Meaning of Existence

Why does anything exist? What is the purpose of life? Is there an underlying reason for the cosmos, or is it a grand accident without design? For millennia, religions and philosophies have offered answers, ranging from divine purpose to absurdity. Cosmologists state if the physical laws (electromagnetic force, the strong and weak nuclear force, and gravity) were changed by less than 1%, then molecules, galaxies, and a planet with life as we know it could not have existed. The universe also appears to have been "**fine-tuned**" since the very moment of creation, causing many to believe this affirms an Intelligent Universe (God) who gives meaning to existence. While each worldview offers insight, no single explanation has laid to rest the ache of this question. The mystery of existence may not be something to solve, but something to live into, moment by moment. As to reality, science explains the **what**; religion offers the **why**.

The Theory of Everything

Physicists continue their quest for a "Theory of Everything"—a single, elegant equation that unites general relativity with quantum mechanics and explains all known forces in the material universe. String theory, loop quantum gravity, and other models strive toward this goal. Yet despite their mathematical beauty, no theory has yet reconciled the divide between the very large (universe) and the very small (quantum sub-atomic particles). The search continues, reflecting our innate longing for coherence, for unity in diversity.

Dark Matter and Dark Energy

Together, dark matter and dark energy make up about 95% of the known universe—yet we cannot see, touch, or directly measure either. We know dark matter exists by its gravitational effects on galaxies. And we infer dark energy through the accelerating expansion of the universe. But their true nature remains unknown. What are these mysterious forces? Are they evidence of new particles or new laws of physics? Or might they point to realities that lie beyond the reach of current scientific tools?

Black Holes

Black holes are regions in space with such strong gravity that nothing, not even light, can escape. They are formed when massive stars collapse at the end of their life cycle. Scientists took the first image of a black hole using Event Horizon Telescope observations of the center of the galaxy M87. The image showed a bright ring formed as light bends in the intense gravity around a black hole that is 6.5 billion times more massive than the Sun. We will speak more to this in later chapters of this book.

Death and the Afterlife

What happens when we die? Does consciousness survive physical death? Are there realms beyond this life? Nearly every culture and spiritual tradition offers some version of life after death—from reincarnation to resurrection to the continuation of the soul. Near-death experiences, past-life memories, and spiritual encounters offer clues, yet definitive answers remain. The mystery of death, like the mystery of birth, invites reverence. It reminds us of our limits, our longings, and our hope.

Paranormal Phenomena

Accounts of apparitions, telepathy, and precognition are found in every culture. While mainstream science often dismisses such reports as anecdotal or unprovable, millions of people report personal experiences that suggest otherwise. **Near-death experiences**, shared death experiences, and inexplicable **synchronicities** challenge the boundaries of what is considered possible. These could be glimpses into dimensions we do not yet understand. Below are books by the J. Newton Rayzor Chair in Philosophy and Religious Thought at Rice University, a friend and respected Professor, Dr. Jeffrey J. Kripal.

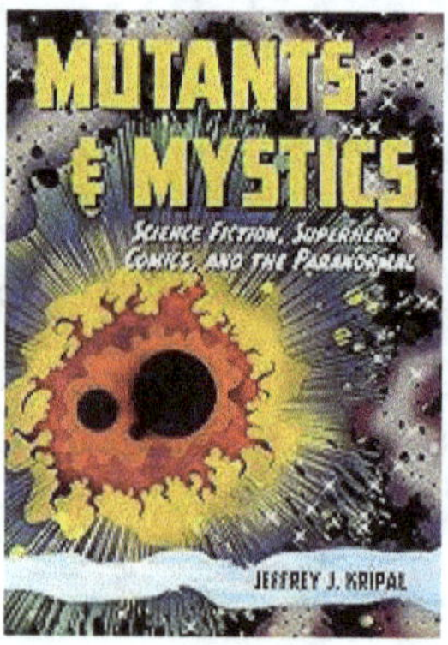

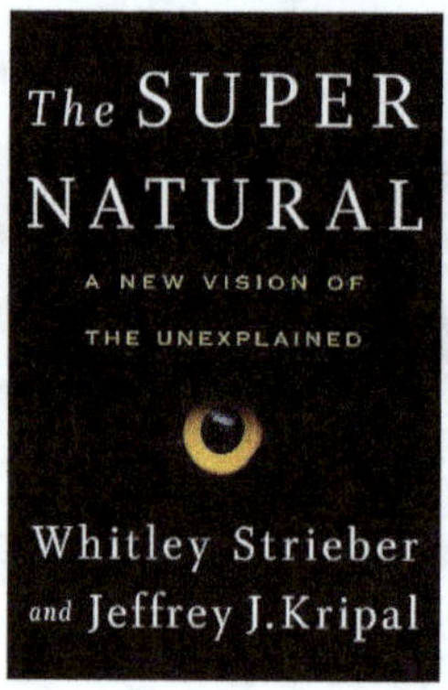

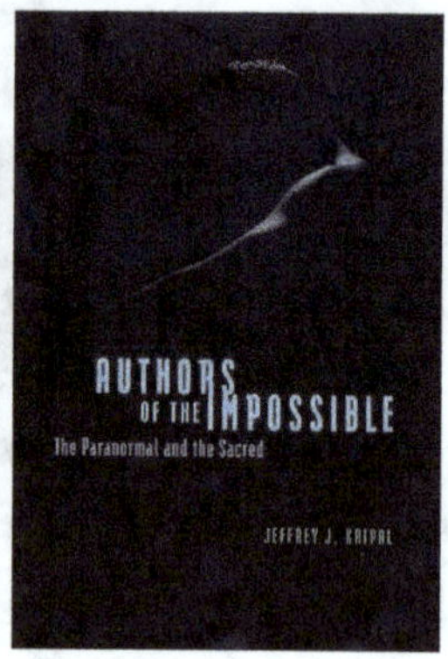

Psychic Phenomena

Closely related to the paranormal, psychic phenomena such as intuition, extrasensory perception (ESP), and an awareness of future events have long fascinated and puzzled researchers. Experiments in remote viewing and mind-matter interaction suggest there may be more to the human mind than neurons firing in the brain. If consciousness extends beyond the physical body, might we all be more interconnected than we imagine?

The Problem of Suffering and Unanswered Prayers

Perhaps no mystery is more personal or more painful than the question of suffering. Why do good people suffer? Why are prayers seemingly ignored? The presence of suffering in a world said to be created by a loving God is one of the oldest and most enduring theological dilemmas. And yet, suffering often becomes the crucible of transformation, awakening compassion, resilience, and insight. Though no answer may fully satisfy, the question itself leads us deeper into the heart of what it means to be human.

Other Great Mysteries

Time and space—what are they, really? Is time linear, cyclical, or an illusion? Do we have free will, or are our lives determined by unseen forces? Is evil a force, a condition, or a necessary contrast to good? These are questions that challenge the limits of our comprehension.

Concluding Comments

As we consider these mysteries, we must acknowledge the limits of our current understanding. Science, philosophy, and spirituality each offer partial insights. The full picture remains hidden, perhaps by design. In the chapters ahead we will explore all of these mysteries which invite us not merely to solve, but to listen deeply, to live with openness and wonder. The path of mystery is not the path of certainty. It is the path of reverence, humility, and trust. As we move forward, may these mysteries not only stimulate our intellect, but open our hearts to the sacred depths of being alive.

> **1 Corinthians 2:9-16**
> But, as it is written, "What no eye has seen, nor ear heard, nor the heart of man imagined, what God has prepared for those who love him"— these things God has revealed to us

> through the Spirit. For the Spirit searches everything, even the depths of God. For who knows a person's thoughts except the spirit of that person, which is in him? So also no one comprehends the thoughts of God except the Spirit of God. Now we have received not the spirit of the world, but the Spirit who is from God, that we might understand the things freely given us by God. And we impart this in words not taught by human wisdom but taught by the Spirit, interpreting spiritual truths to those who are spiritual."

Consciousness and Mindfulness

Mindfulness, as a central practice in Buddhism, involves being present in the moment and observing one's experiences without judgment. It's a key element in developing insight and cultivating a more balanced and peaceful mind.

The Four Foundations of Mindfulness

The Satipatthana Sutta outlines four specific areas for practicing mindfulness:

Body: Paying attention to physical sensations, postures, and movements.

Feelings: Observing the range of emotions, including pleasant, unpleasant, and neutral feelings.

Mind: Noting the nature of mental states, thoughts, and intentions.

Dhammas: Reflecting on the nature of mental phenomena, including the five aggregates (form, feeling, perception, mental formations, and consciousness).

Before moving on to the next chapter you may wish to consider the following questions as you reflect on what we covered in this chapter on the great mysteries of life.

- *Did one or more of the Great Mysteries of Life grip you deeply? What was that like?*
- *Have you been exposed to a paranormal experience? Did you feel comfortable to share your experience with others?*
- *Has the reality of suffering and evil concerned you or touched the life of those you love? If so, the next chapter will address these issues.*

Chapter 9—Mystery of Suffering and Evil

"The evil that is in the world always comes of ignorance..."
—Albert Camus, The Plague

Across cultures and centuries, one question has lingered like a shadow across the human soul:

Why does suffering and evil exist?

Whether encountered as moral wrongdoing, natural disaster, or inner torment, suffering demands an explanation. For those who believe in a just and loving God, it presents a crisis of faith. For others, it points to the enigma of human nature, or the chaos woven into creation itself.

This chapter explores diverse beliefs about the source of suffering and evil—not to resolve the mystery, but to offer insight into the ways people of faith, reason, and lived experience have grappled with this enduring dilemma.

In our bereavement group, I've witnessed this anguish. A mother lost her 29-year-old son suddenly to a fentanyl overdose. Her dream of him marrying and having children were gone in a moment. Another lost her child to murder. Yes, murder. A young woman, raising two children, lost her husband to a fatal motorcycle accident caused by another driver's reckless road rage. Through her tears, we all asked with her: "Why did God let this happen?"

Let us begin with a question we have all heard expressed:

> "How can I believe in an all-powerful God who allows evil to happen every day?"

Why Does God Permit Suffering?

When a child dies, a nation is invaded, or cancer takes hold of a loved one, the heart protests—not only in pain but in outrage. The cry goes out not just for healing, but for understanding.

Blaming God is not just philosophical—it is emotional, existential, relational. For those raised to trust in a God who is both powerful and good, the presence of suffering feels like betrayal. They want to know why God let this happen. The ancient lament of Job still rings true:

> *"Though I cry, 'Violence!' I get no response; though I call for help, there is no justice."*—Job 19:7

This is the problem of evil. The philosopher Epicurus captured its tension in three enduring questions:

- If God is willing to prevent evil but not able, is He not omnipotent?
- If He is able but not willing, is He not good?
- If He is both willing and able, why does evil exist?

The attempt to reconcile God's goodness with the existence of evil is called **theodicy**. The word comes from theos meaning God and dike meaning justice. Christian thinkers like Augustine and Aquinas argued that free will is necessary for love and virtue—but it also opens the door to suffering. C.S. Lewis described pain as "God's megaphone" to get our attention. Theologian and Philosopher of Religion, John Hick, has proposed suffering is part of a soul-making journey.

And yet when in grief, a theodicy explanation can feel cold. As Rabbi Harold Kushner wrote in *When Bad Things Happen to Good People*: "People don't want theological explanations. They want to know someone understands what they're going through."

Rightly understood, to cry out against God is a form of faith. Lament itself is a sacred act—a protest of love. As the mystics and Hebrew psalmists teach, sorrow can become a kind of worship when it is laid bare before the Divine.

In the Christian tradition, God does not remain removed from suffering. Through the Incarnation, God enters it. On the Cross, Jesus cried out: *"My God, my God, why have you forsaken me?"* (Mark 15:34). This is not a God above evil, but a God within it—who weeps, bleeds, and walks with us through the valley of shadow.

World Religions on Evil

Judaism and Christianity: The Fall and the Freedom to Choose
In Genesis, evil enters the world not with malice, but with a choice. Adam and Eve's desire for autonomy leads to alienation. Augustine called this disobedience original sin and defined evil as a turning from God's light. Saint Irenaeus later suggested that suffering has a redemptive function—it shapes and strengthens the soul. Yet many still can ask:

> *"What did I do wrong? I've tried to live a good life. Why did God let this happen?"*

Christian
In an article on the Science of Evil and the Theology of Evil (2019), Lutheran Emeritus Professor of Theology, Ted Peters, mentions Sociobiologist Edward O. Wilson who observes that the **Golden Rule** "is perhaps the only precept found in all organized religions, and The Rule is fundamental for all moral reasoning." He quotes Jesus in his Sermon on the Mountain where he says: "In everything do unto others what you would have them to do you, for this sums up the Law and the Prophets" (Matthew 7:12; Luke 6:31). Peters says Martin Luther has said The Golden Rule agrees with natural law.

Islam: Evil as Test and Temptation
In Islam, evil is part of the divine test. Iblis (Satan), who refused to bow to Adam, tempts humanity—but cannot force it. The Qur'an emphasizes human responsibility and the inner struggle with the nafs—the lower self.

> *"The greatest jihad is against the self."—The Prophet Muhammad*

Here, evil is not a cosmic enemy, but a spiritual challenge meant to refine the soul.

Hinduism and Buddhism: Ignorance, Attachment, and Illusion
In many Eastern traditions, evil arises from ignorance (avidya) and attachment (tanha). Hinduism teaches that the soul is divine but forgets its unity with all things. This forgetfulness breeds suffering.

In Buddhism, evil is not an external force but a distortion of perception. The "three poisons"—attachment (greed), anger (hatred), and ignorance (delusion)—obscure our awareness, causing pain and suffering.

Philosophical Beliefs: The Free Will Defense

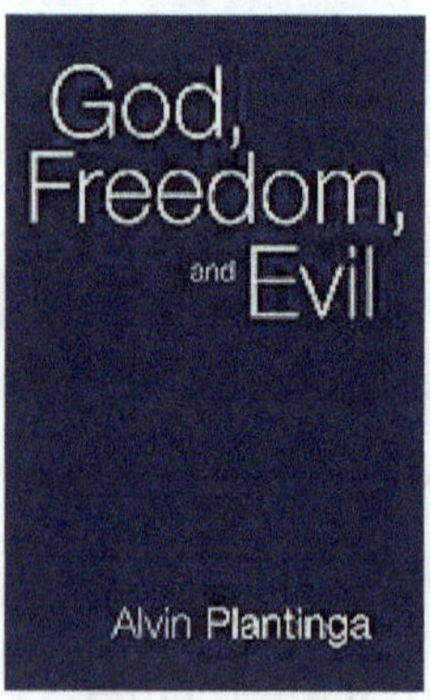

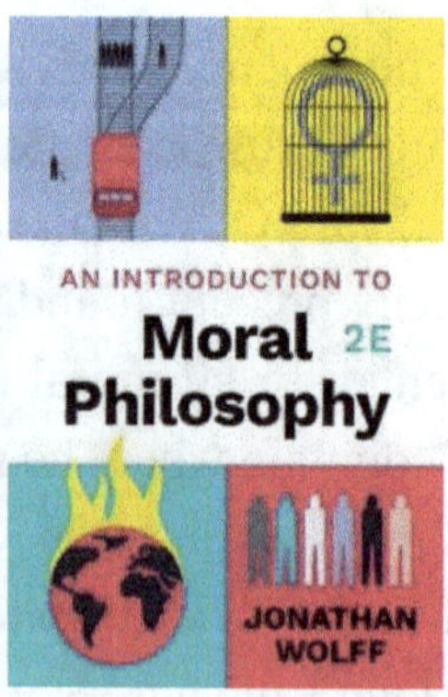

Alvin Plantinga's Free Will Defense

The challenge of evil has long occupied philosophers. In *God, Freedom, and Evil,* Alvin Plantinga (1989) defends the fact that God created human beings with a free will which means they can do good or evil. The fact that free creatures can go wrong, however, Plantinga says, counts neither against God's omnipotence nor against His goodness; for God could only have prevented the occurrence of moral evil by removing the possibility of moral good. Plantinga says **free will is essential** to love and virtue, and worth the risk of its misuse.

De Florio & Frigerio (2013) have written a strong challenge to Plantinga's defense of God.

Psychological Perspectives: The Shadow and Dehumanization

Dehumanization

In his book, *Less Than Human: Why We Demonize, Enslave, and Exterminate Others* (2011), David Livingston explains how dehumanization enables atrocity. He argues that dehumanization is not merely a product of propaganda or hatred, but a deep-seated cognitive habit humans have yielded to throughout our evolutionary and cultural history. From slavery and genocide (The Holocaust) to modern **hate speech**, Smith shows how perpetrators suspend empathy by **labeling** others as animals, vermin, demons, or worse. It is a way nations activate their citizens and soldiers when at war. Today, demeaning slanders and **dehumanizing words** are used by candidates running for political office and we elect them routinely!

This is an ever-present danger in our world today, in political rhetoric and cultural divisions.

Freud and Jung

Freud viewed aggression as part of the psyche's inner conflict. Jung offered a more spiritual insight—evil arises from the Shadow, the denied part of ourselves. Healing begins with self-awareness and inner integration. *"Knowing your own darkness is the best method for dealing with the darkness of other people."*—C. G. Jung

To Jung, confronting the **Shadow** is a path to wholeness. Evil is not eradicated, but integrated through self-awareness, humility, and spiritual work.

Scientific Views: Evolution, Brain, and Behavior

From a biological perspective, "evil" behaviors often reflect ancient survival mechanisms—tribalism, competition, dominance.

In award-winning British researcher, Simon Baron-Cohen's book, *The Science of Evil: On Empathy and the Origins of Cruelty* (2011) the author looks at Borderline Personality Disorder, Narcissism, and psychosis which have one thing in common—**lack of empathy**. He also recognizes in all people social and environmental factors can erode empathy leading to neglect and abuse. Neuroscience also shows how damage to the brain can impair empathy, suggesting that moral behavior is at least partly physiological.

A Darwinian Approach to Evil

Kjeldgaard-Christiansen (2016) says the concept of evil is so problematic that philosophers and theologians have offered different and often contradictory ideas about evil for thousands of years. He says social psychologists have taken the easy route by saying: "People are bad because they are bad." The author argues that evolved cognitive dispositions inform the archetypical villain of popular literature, film and video games. He suggests there may be an adaptive function to this fictional villain space which allows society to affirm by contrast its prosocial values. Kjeldgaard-Christiansen proposes a "**poetics of evil**" that is integrated with the sciences of the human mind. From a Darwinian perspective, evil has its adaptive roots that licenses violence and devastating punishment.

Integrating Darwinian evolution with the notion of evil, Kjeldgaard-Christiansen says that like other primates, humans evolved to live and thrive in cooperative groups. Moral behavior was built on kin selection and reciprocal altruism. Over time, as societies grew larger, people no longer know each other and adapted an attitude to always be **selfish** (caring only for those in one's own house). He says this logic is captured by the concept of **welfare tradeoff ratios** (WTR) that govern how we treat others and how they are to treat us. Of course, humans also made adaptations to ensure cooperation does not encourage free-loaders, antisocial individualists, and competing coalitions. He says our universal conception of evil is one such adaptation and, from this perspective, evil is a designation reserved for those who have a sustained mismatch between the expected welfare tradeoffs we grant for ourselves and those in our group. Finally, he says evil seems to bear a relation to **disgust**—we find disgusting people immoral, and we find immoral people disgusting.

Yet the brain is plastic. Compassion and empathy can be cultivated. Biology is not our destiny.

Concluding Comments: The Mystery that Binds All Beliefs

The source of evil cannot be reduced to a single cause. From Satan to Shadow, from *Iblis* to ignorance, beliefs about evil reflect our deepest fears—and highest hopes. They tell us about the nature of God, the limits of freedom, the depth of the human heart, and the mystery of existence itself.

Then why is there suffering and illness? Buddhism views suffering as a school—without the experience of pain, consciousness cannot develop, just as muscles grown under strain, so the spirit is strengthened through the rough time. Each life is a lesson. Even the hardest destinies have a purpose, though the human mind cannot always understand it. When we leave this place, much will become clear, and then we will understand no one has ever truly been alone.

Have you struggled with why there is suffering and evil in the world. Why does God permit evil and suffering?

Yet amid these differences, a common call emerges: **to resist, to awaken, to heal**. Evil may be mystery—but goodness is a miracle. And every belief that wrestles with darkness does so because it seeks the light.

Ponder that thought as we prepare to enter Chapter 10: The Sacred and Missing Link. Which, because evil will remain during this lifetime, we must learn how to embrace spirituality and to be aware that God is always present especially in our moments of suffering. But first, consider also these important questions:

- *Alvin Plantinga's Theodicy is a defense of God creating human beings with a* ***free will****. Do you agree that humanity should have the freedom to do what is good and what is evil?*
- *David L. Smith talks about* ***dehumanization*** *in his book. What do you think about his explanation as to why cultures and nations demonize, enslave, and exterminate others?*
- *Have you heard dehumanization language used in everyday conversations? At political or religious gatherings? On social media sites, in movies, art, or music?*

Chapter 10—The Sacred and the Missing Link

In every ancient culture, the sacred was central. It imbued the natural world, shaped the structure of society, and infused daily rituals with meaning. Myths, sacred texts, and spiritual practices served not only to explain the origins of life and the universe but also to offer guidance, protection, and identity. Sacred sites—whether temples, burial grounds, or places of pilgrimage—acted as portals to something beyond the material, drawing people into community, remembrance, and reverence.

Stonehenge

Decades ago, my wife and I took our five children on a trip to England and Scotland. One of the highpoints of the trip was viewing Stonehenge, where we stood in silence with others, aware this was a sacred space. We were told the space was first used as a burial ground, attesting to the fact that they too grieved the death of their loved ones. The stones came later, perhaps 2,500 years ago, and we tried to imagine how thousands of years ago people could have moved those massive stones into place. Each of the great stones stand silently, reverently, and collectively to honor those who had gone before. Stonehenge was a very memorable and moving experience.

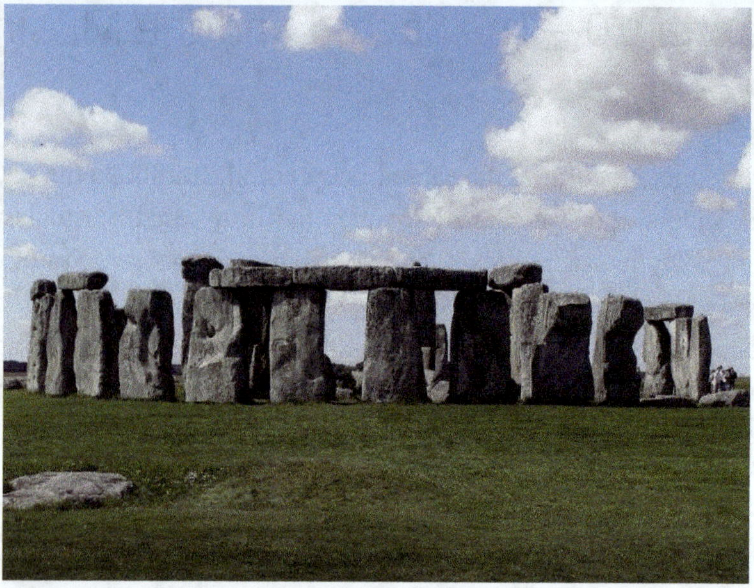

Stonehenge. Picture by Gareth Wiscombe, Public Domain licensed under the Creative Commons Attribution 2.0 Generic license. Wikimedia Commons.

Ancient rituals and sacred places offered something modern society often struggles to maintain: a deep sense of connection—to one another, to our ancestors, and to something greater than ourselves. The sacred offered meaning during suffering and served as a wellspring for hope.

Something is Missing

In our modern world, many people feel that something essential has been lost. The once-vibrant connection to the sacred has been eroded by materialism, secularism, and a growing reliance on empirical science as the sole arbiter of truth. This disconnection from the sacred has led to a deep existential emptiness, a spiritual homelessness that separates the individual and collective soul.

Carl Jung addressed "the spiritual problem of modern man" in his 1928 *Collected Works, Volume 10*. He wrote:

> I realize only too well that my faith in the rational organization of the world—that old dream of the millennium when peace and harmony reign—has grown pale… Science has long ago torn this lovely veil to shreds… Through his skepticism modern man is thrown back on himself.
> Modern mankind has lost all the metaphysical certainties of his medieval brother and set up in their place the ideals of material security, general welfare and humanitarianism

What, then, is the sacred? In truth, the sacred is not confined to organized religion. Rather, religions point beyond to that which is sacred—the divine, the quality we feel when confronted by awe—in nature, in beauty, in birth and death, in love, and in mystery. The sacred invites us to step beyond the ego, to feel ourselves as part of something vast and interconnected, connected to the Ultimate Source, the Absolute, God.

Sacred Rituals

For me, the sense of sacredness came alive in the rituals of the Episcopal Church. I was raised in a Protestant church that emphasized only baptism among the practices of ritual. Later in life, when I was exposed to the Episcopal Church, I came to value and appreciate its liturgy, which was inherited from the Church of England and Catholicism. I loved the three-year cycle of prayers and scriptural readings found in the *Book of Common Prayer*, and the six liturgical seasons—Advent, Christmas, Epiphany, Lent, Easter, and Pentecost.

None is more special than Holy Week, which begins with Palm Sunday when Jesus rode into Jerusalem on a donkey, with crowds waving palm branches and shouting their Hosannas. And, on Palm Sunday we Episcopalians enter the church waving palm branches. Then the liturgy shifts as we shout, "Crucify him! Crucify him!" We do this to acknowledge Jesus went to the Cross because of our sin as well as the sin of all humanity. Daily liturgies carry us down the road to Maundy Thursday when Jesus is arrested and thrown into prison, followed by what is called "Good Friday" when Jesus is crucified. We spend Holy Saturday in silence as we ponder that Jesus died for the sin of the world. Then on Easter morning, everything changes to a celebration of the Resurrection. These rituals provide a path for our journey with the Divine, reminding us of something timeless and true.

Sharing the story of Jesus' death requires me to pause for a clarification. It would be easy to say Jews in the first century crucified Jesus. But, rightly understood, Christianity proclaims that Jesus was crucified because of the sin of the world (everyone's sin, your sin, and my sin). The human choice to turn from our creator is the reason Jesus died on the Cross, not merely because he was rejected by the Pharisees, Sadducees, and people of his day. Had Jesus not died God's plan of redemption would not have taken place. In the garden before his death, Jesus asked his heavenly Father to save him from what he knew would soon take place. Then he said, "But not my will but Thy will be done."

As hard as it is to understand, Christianity says it was God the Father who sent God the Son to die by crucifixion, not the Israelites. The Christian story is God chose to incarnate in a Jew, Jesus, to bring about redemption and to reconcile all people unto Himself. In Jesus' death, God was saying, "I love you enough to die for you." The fact is, if Jesus had not died and had lived to old age, there would have been no resurrection and Christianity would never have formed as we know it. It was the resurrection of Christ that galvanized the apostles and the early church. Without Jesus' death and resurrection, God's plan of redemption would not have taken place. If anything, Jewish people should be appreciated. After all, Jesus was born, raised, and died a Jew. There is absolutely no basis for antisemitism if you accept the Christian message. Jesus loved his Jewish friends and neighbors, and we should too.

While many love liturgy and rituals, others seek the sacred in silence, in meditation, in the stillness of nature, in the stirring notes of music, or in the quiet brushstrokes of art. To recover a sense of the sacred in our modern lives does not require a return to dogma. Rather, it calls for awareness of wonder and a renewed openness to the mysteries that surround us.

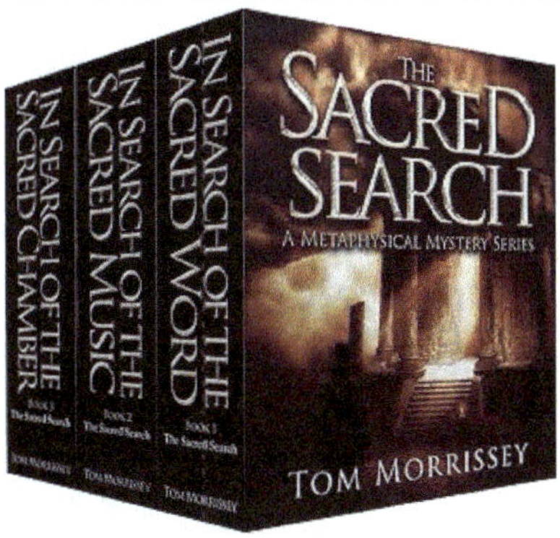

The Arts and The Sacred

In his book, *The Power of Art*, Simon Schama asks a provocative question in his chapter on the artist Jacques-Louis David:

> If art can make you happy, can it also make you good? If it can move you to ecstasy or tears, should it also move you to be a stand-up citizen? Can modern secular painting have the conversionary power of Christian masterpieces: the power to save souls, not from sin, but from selfishness? Ought the power of art lend itself to the art of power?

To all these questions, Schama says Jacques-Louis David replied with an adamant yes. Perhaps this is the missing link we are called to rediscover. In a world saturated with data but starved for meaning, we must once again learn to recognize and honor the sacred—not only in temples and scriptures, but in the natural world, in shared rituals, in the arts, in the human body, and in the enduring mysteries of life itself.

The Sacred Beckons

In every age, the sacred has beckoned us beyond the surface of things—calling us to pause, to remember, to feel, and to belong. Whether through ancient stones aligned with the stars, communal rituals passed down through centuries, or the quiet ache of longing for something more, the sacred has never disappeared. It has only gone into hiding, waiting for us to recover the eyes to see it.

We live in a world rich with information but often starved for meaning. In the rush of progress, we may have lost our footing in mystery. Yet mystery has not forsaken us. It waits in the silence between words, the stillness of a morning, the brushstroke of a painting, or the hush of holy week on bended knee.

In an essay entitled, *Beyond materialism: A Pan-Spiritist Perspective*, Stephen Taylor, Ph.D., says "The materialist model does not explain the world very well." He continues, "But if you replace the materialist model of science with the idea that the ground of reality of the universe is a spiritual force—a fundamental consciousness or spirit—then everything begins to make more sense."

However, rather than attempting to replace the materialist model with a spiritual one, I believe there is a way to **embrace both** science and the sacred (as I have in my own life). Yet the challenge is great. Quantum physicist and theologian John Polkinghorne (2007) writes:

> Science plays an influential role in contemporary thinking, both through content of its actual discoveries and through its style of evidence-based thinking. If religion is to retain credibility, it must find a voice that is audible in the

intellectual setting. Today vigorous activity is taking place across the science and religion frontier. However, the attempt to integrate these two great aspects of human inquiry is not just a current concern, for it has a long history.

Science, Nature, and the Sacred

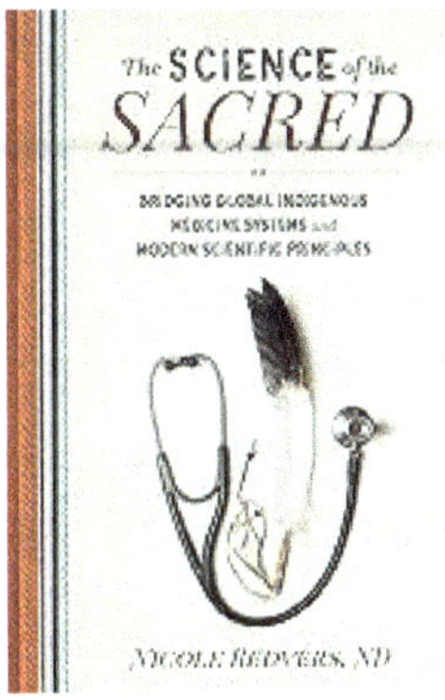

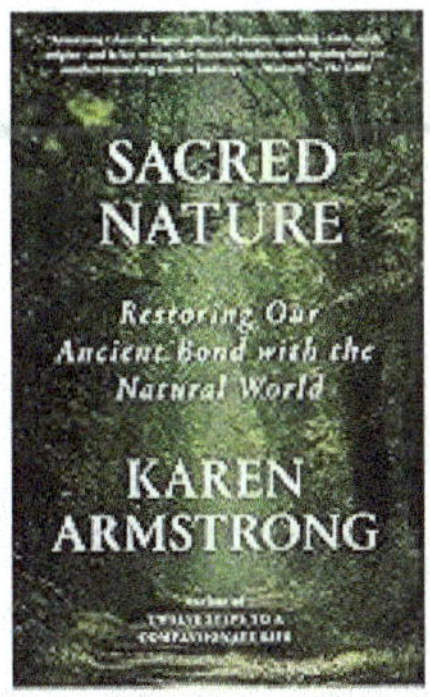

Science, nature, and the sacred—all three are essential to adequately embrace our understanding the world and our place in it. Through empirical observation and experimentation, science provides a framework for understanding the natural world, while nature includes all living and non-living aspects of scientific inquiry. The sacred, often associated with spiritual or religious experiences, can be seen as a way of experiencing the awe and wonder of both science and nature, while potentially revealing a deeper meaning or connection to the universe.

Indian-born mathematician, statistician, and Colorado State University professor emeritus, Jagdish Srivastava (1933-2010), is author of the book, *A Viable New Paradigm for Quantum Reality* (2011), which provides a solution to some of the major controversies raging in the field of physics. The author relates that he had the "thrill" of being a scientist who loved to argue that God does not exist. However, over time he came to see imitations with his "cherished deity," science. In 1960, he "temporarily quit physics and logic." He explains what happened next:

> Shyly, hesitantly at first, I began to embrace spirituality, which to me was the attitude that reality would lead one to. **I saw that reality had no horizons**; I decided to let myself go wherever it leads me. I decided to dedicate myself to research on science and spirituality. Science does not stand in contradiction to spirituality; the former is a tiny and important part of the latter.

To make the transition that allowed him to integrate science and spirituality, Srivastava found a new reality unfolded for him when he gave up the "luggage" of attachments, aversions and selfish world desires. He found the benefit of incorporating spirituality to be great: "For what one acquires on the spiritual path cannot be even dreamt of by those who have not experienced it. Indeed, consciousness increases, leading to a very changed perspective and to new abilities."

Restoring a sense of the sacred in our lives does not require the rejection of reason but to welcome wonder. It is to open ourselves to that which cannot be measured but can be known in the depths of our being. The sacred is not merely a message from the past—it is a path to our spiritual home.

Concluding Comments

As we move now into the next chapter, we turn toward the greatest mystery of all: the mystery of God. Throughout history, humanity has wrestled with the divine—with awe, with longing, with love, and with fear. Every culture has given voice to this longing in prayers, in poems, in sacred texts, and in silence. But who—or what—is God? Is the Divine a person, a presence, a force? A Creator, a Consciousness, an eternal pulse of love?

Is God knowable? Or is God the great unknowable—forever beyond our grasp, yet closer to us than our breath? What do you think?

In Chapter 11, The God Mystery, we will step into this sacred terrain. Not to define God, for the mystery of God may not be something we solve, but something we enter—with reverence, humility, and a heart wide open.

A few questions before moving on may be appropriate:

- *Have you experienced a sacred space in nature or at a site of worship or burial ground?*
- *Many have encountered the divine in rituals. Has that been your experience?*
- *Do you believe there is a way to embrace* ***both*** *science and the sacred?*

Chapter 11—The God Mystery

The Hidden and the Near

God is, by nature, a mystery—not because God is unknowable, but because the Infinite cannot be fully grasped by the finite. God is both **transcendent**, existing beyond space, time, and human categories, and **immanent**, closer to us than our very breath. We cannot see or touch God directly with our five senses, yet many of us have sensed the Divine in the beauty of creation, in the compassion of another person, or in a sudden, inward clarity when spiritually awakened.

Pope Paul VI described divine mystery as "a reality imbued with the hidden presence of God." This is not a puzzle to be solved, but a **presence to be encountered**—a truth we grow into through awe, openness, and experience. In fact, the very language we use to describe God often falters. The more we speak, the more we realize: the Mystery exceeds our words.

Modern science, too, hints at **unseen dimensions**—realms of energy, consciousness, and information beyond the senses. Quantum physicists speak of the "virtual" field that existed before the Big Bang. Could this be the sacred ground beneath all that is—the silent source of life and love?

While transcendent, the mystery of God is also profoundly intimate. Through prayer, meditation, worship, and stillness, many report feeling **seen, known, and guided**. This knowing is not the product of logical reasoning, but something deeper—an intuition of the heart, a spiritual perception.

The Inward Experience

Years ago, my wife and I bought a new home. Before moving in, I dropped by the house to inspect progress with updates to the house.

Suddenly, my next-door neighbor appeared, introduced himself, and said, "I hear you are a Christian." I said, "Yes sir, that is true." He then said, "This morning while I was shaving, I heard, 'Why do you honor me on Sundays but deny me the rest of the week?' What do you think?" I said, "Let's put it to the test. I don't believe you would say that about yourself, nor do I believe the enemy of your soul would say that either. So, I believe God has spoken to you." My neighbor appeared stricken and asked, "What should I do?"

I said, "I'm not going to tell you what to do, but why don't you pray and ask God what you are to do." He prayed and was convicted that he had been writing contracts that favored his clients. Making a change meant that very day my neighbor lost his largest client, but thereafter his other clients knew they could trust him in all things. My neighbor's business grew and prospered with over fifty employees. He frequently shares with others the story of his encounter with God that changed his life.

The Christian Mystery: Incarnation

One of the most profound Christian expressions of divine mystery is the Incarnation—the belief that God entered human life in the person of Jesus of Nazareth. Fully human and fully Divine, Jesus offers a window into the very heart of God: not a distant judge but a compassionate, healing presence. In Jesus the invisible becomes visible. The unknowable has chosen to be known.

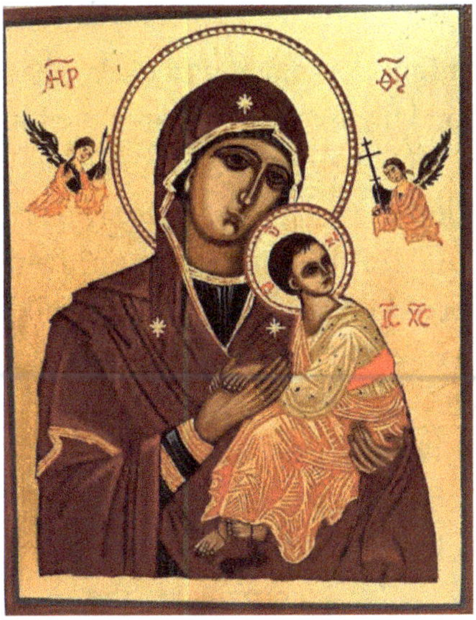

The Virgin of Passion
"Theotokos"
The Mother of God

Icon written by Fr. John Graham at an Icon Writing Workshop held at St. Martin's Episcopal Church, Houston, Texas on March 19-23, 2007. Teacher: Theresa Harrison of Jacksonville, Florida.

Today, there are scientists who describe the Big Bang as the "Big Breath" to refer to Consciousness being the source of creation of the universe. They also believe that the Absolute has been continuously present since creation—in every aspect of the unfolding of creation. The Church and its sacraments also point to mystery. In water, bread, wine, and word, something more than symbol is at work. Christians believe the hidden Presence of God is encountered through these sacred signs—not apart from, but within the physical world. This intertwining of spirit and matter speaks to the core message of Christianity and all world religions: God's love made real.

Divine Mystery Across the World Religions

A Personal Awakening. For much of my life, I had little exposure to faith traditions beyond my own. Raised in a predominantly Christian community, I knew of Judaism but had never met a rabbi or studied other religions in depth with an open heart. That changed when I became President of the Institute for Spirituality and Health in Houston. A Hindu board member invited me to his home for dinner. I assumed I would speak about the Institute's mission. Instead, after my arrival, I was asked to share my personal faith story. I swallowed hard and said, "Are you sure you want me to share my faith story?" Yes, I was told, that was what they wanted to hear.

Surprised but willing, I shared my Christian journey and my spiritual awakening. To my amazement, the men around the table nodded with deep resonance—and then, one by one, shared their stories of encountering God. Their words echoed my own experience. I left that evening both humbled and awakened—not only to the prejudice of my former assumptions, but to the truth I had always suspected in my heart: that **God has reached out to all people**, across every culture and faith tradition, throughout human history.

Psychologist and theologian William James spoke of "one goal, many paths." James' work affirmed the richness of religious diversity and the essential unity of spiritual longing.

Judaism

Judaism reveres God as beyond name or form—and yet intimately involved in human history. The Hebrew name for God, YHWH, often pronounced "Yahweh," traditionally is not spoken by Jews as a sign of reverence. God speaks through prophets, calls people to justice and mercy, and establishes a sacred covenant with the people of Israel. Despite immense suffering, including the Holocaust and ongoing antisemitism, Judaism continues to affirm the faithfulness of God.

Islam

In Islam, Allah is both utterly beyond and intimately near—"closer than our jugular vein," as the Qur'an says. The 99 Names of God offer poetic glimpses of the divine character: The Merciful, The Compassionate, The Sustainer. Muslims are called to submit to God's will, to live in peace and justice, and to remember that unity is at the heart of all things.

Hinduism

Hindus see Brahman as the ultimate reality—both immanent and transcendent—made known through a rich tapestry of deities like Vishnu, Shiva, and Lakshmi. These expressions help followers relate to different facets of the divine. Ancient texts such as the Bhagavad Gita and the Upanishads resonate with many modern seekers, especially as quantum physics echoes their themes of interconnectedness and unseen reality (Prabhupada, 1983).

Buddhism

Though often described as not a religion, Buddhism embraces temples, rituals, sacred writings, feast days, ordained clergy, monastic settings, reincarnation, and a reverence for the mystery of being. The ultimate aim is enlightenment—perceiving life in its true essence. The teachings of Buddha on interdependence, impermanence, and mindfulness as a way to liberation. The Dharmakaya, is sometimes viewed as the infinite ground of being—a reality beyond form.

Taoism

Rooted in ancient China, Taoism speaks of the Tao—the Way—the source and flow of all life. The Tao cannot be fully described, only lived. It teaches harmony, balance, and surrender to the rhythms of nature and mystery.

Indigenous Traditions

In Indigenous spiritualities, the divine is felt through nature, ancestors, and sacred ritual. The Great Spirit or Creator is present in wind and stone, fire and water. Spirituality is not separated from daily life, but woven into it—honored through dance, story, and reverence for the earth.

Agnostics, Atheists, and their Unnamed Longing

Even those who do not claim a formal belief in God—agnostics, atheists, secular humanists—often encounter moments of mystery. A sense of awe at a newborn's cry, a star-filled sky, or the death of a loved one may provoke questions about consciousness, love, and eternity.

Though some may argue that science has rejected God, others among them recognize a hunger for meaning and beauty that scientific facts and theories cannot satisfy. In moments of grief, wonder, or deep relationship, they too may sense what they cannot name—a longing that transcends explanation.

The Golden Rule: A Shared Thread

Across these varied traditions runs a common thread—The Golden Rule: Do unto others as you would have them do unto you. This universal ethic reminds us that while names and doctrines differ, love, compassion, and humility are shared across humanity. A photograph of the Golden Rule is found at the end of this chapter.

Science and the Sacred Unknown

From Big Bang to Big Mystery

Science once tried to keep God at a distance. But in recent decades, that division has softened. The more we learn, the more we discover how much we cannot explain.

The **Big Bang** itself begins in mystery—an explosion of light and energy from what? From where? From a hidden field of potentiality? I and others call it the "Big Breath." Respected physicists like Paul Davies have suggested that the fine-tuning of the universe implies a kind of intelligence—perhaps not a personal God, but a conscious order behind all things.

Quantum Physics and Consciousness.

Quantum physics adds to the wonder. Particles exist as **probabilities** due to quantum uncertainty until an "interaction" takes place resulting in a single outcome. Reality, it seems, is relational—and consciousness might be a creative force. Physicist John Wheeler once said, "We are not simply observers; we are participants in bringing the universe into being." Could this be the edge where science meets spirituality? We will explore the quantum reality in chapters ahead.

The Human Brain and Transcendence

Neuroscience has mapped the brain during prayer, meditation, and mystical states. Dr. Andrew Newberg found that spiritual practices activate regions associated with compassion, attention, and joy. Rather than disproving faith, these studies suggest that **our brains are wired for connection**—with each other and perhaps with something beyond.

The Dance of Order and Emergence

From ecosystems to human culture, science reveals patterns of cooperation, beauty, and emergence. This is not randomness, but deep structure—**a creative unfolding that invites reverence**.

As Pascal once wrote, the God of spiritual experience is not merely the "god of the philosophers," but the Living God—the God who meets us in awe, silence, and surrender.

Concluding Comments

Whether through sacred texts or subatomic mysteries, whether called God, Allah, Brahman, the Tao, or simply **the Mystery**, something calls to us—**beyond explanation, yet intimately near**. In every tradition, in every honest heart, the path begins with humility and a willingness to listen.

As we turn now to Chapter 12: Spiritual Practices for Navigating Mystery, we will explore how we open ourselves to this Mystery—through prayer, meditation, silence, service, ritual, and presence. These are the tools of spiritual perception—the ways we train the soul to see what cannot be seen with the eyes alone. Let us continue this journey—not to solve the Mystery, but to walk more deeply into it.

On the following page view the image of **The Golden Rule** which—presented in the words of the world's major religions—hangs in our office at the Institute for Spirituality and Health in Houston. It is a visual reminder that we are not as divided as we may think. It is depicted here with permission of its creator, Paul McKenna, who provided the poster which follows. I encourage you to read through this depiction prayerfully as there is much to learn and be edified.

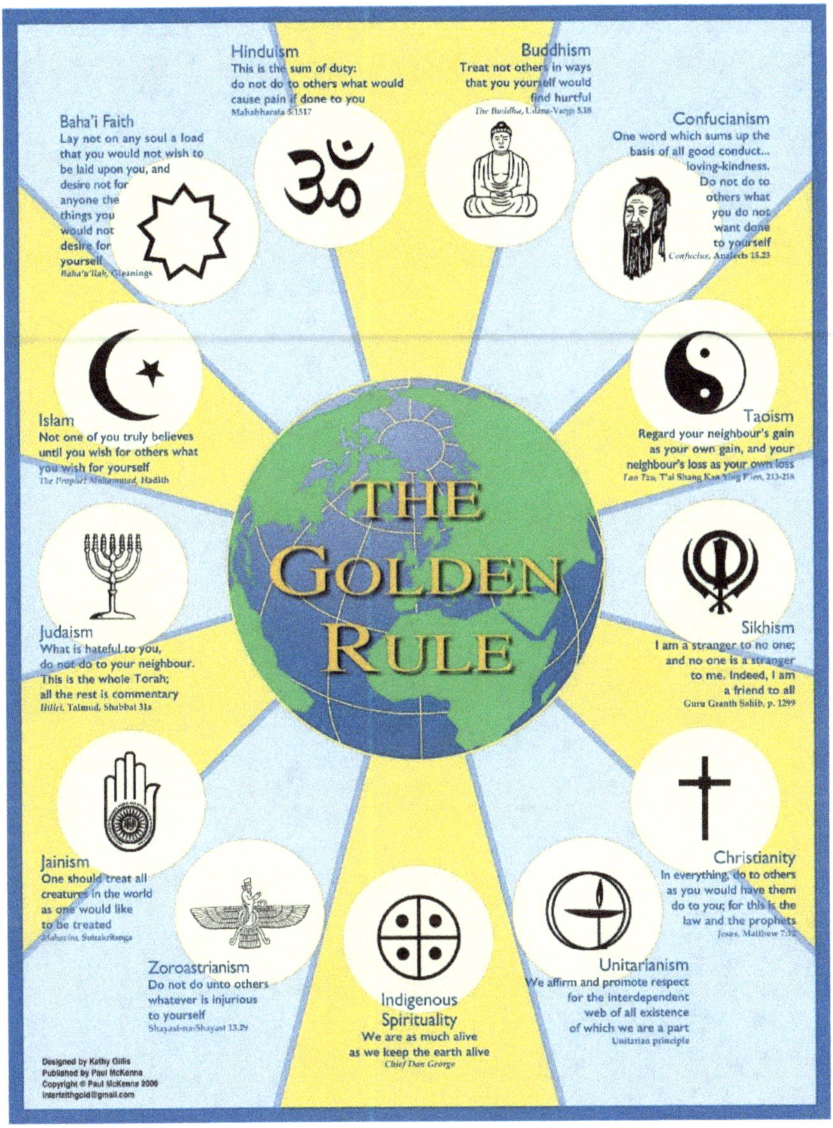
THE GOLDEN RULE
Hinduism
This is the sum of duty: do not do to others what would cause pain if done to you
Mahabharata 5:1517
Buddhism
Treat not others in ways that you yourself would find hurtful
The Buddha, Udana-Varga 5.18
Baha'i Faith
Lay not on any soul a load that you would not wish to be laid upon you, and desire not for anyone the things you would not desire for yourself
Baha'u'llah, Gleanings
Confucianism
One word which sums up the basis of all good conduct... loving-kindness. Do not do to others what you do not want done to yourself
Confucius, Analects 15.23
Islam
Not one of you truly believes until you wish for others what you wish for yourself
The Prophet Muhammad, Hadith
Taoism
Regard your neighbour's gain as your own gain, and your neighbour's loss as your own loss
Lao Tzu, T'ai Shang Kan Ying P'ien, 213-218
Judaism
What is hateful to you, do not do to your neighbour. This is the whole Torah; all the rest is commentary
Hillel, Talmud, Shabbat 31a
Sikhism
I am a stranger to no one; and no one is a stranger to me. Indeed, I am a friend to all
Guru Granth Sahib, p. 1299
Jainism
One should treat all creatures in the world as one would like to be treated
Mahavira, Sutrakritanga
Christianity
In everything, do to others as you would have them do to you; for this is the law and the prophets
Jesus, Matthew 7:12
Zoroastrianism
Do not do unto others whatever is injurious to yourself
Shayast-na-Shayast 13.29
Indigenous Spirituality
We are as much alive as we keep the earth alive
Chief Dan George
Unitarianism
We affirm and promote respect for the interdependent web of all existence of which we are a part
Unitarian principle
Designed by Kathy Gillis
Published by Paul McKenna
Copyright © Paul McKenna 2000
interfaithgold@gmail.com

Chapter 12—Spiritual Practices for Navigating Mystery

Embracing Mystery

In a world that values certainty, the invitation to dwell in mystery can feel unsettling—even risky. Yet the great spiritual traditions teach us that mystery is not something to solve, but something to embrace. Mystery humbles the intellect, softens the heart, and opens the spirit to a deeper awareness of reality. It is in this liminal space—between knowing and unknowing—that the soul awakens.

To navigate mystery is not to flee from uncertainty but to live in it with courage and grace. Here, spiritual practices become essential—not as answers, but as companions, guideposts, and nourishment. These practices do not dispel mystery; they invite us to live more deeply within it.

1. Acceptance of Uncertainty

The first and perhaps most difficult spiritual practice is simply this: to accept that we do not—and cannot—know everything. This is not resignation, but release. It is the sacred art of surrendering control and living with wonder. Acceptance opens the door to faith, humility, and trust. It is the soil in which awe can grow.

Buddhism teaches, "Don't worry, be present." Our mind fears illusions while our spirit finds peace in presence. Meditation practices across traditions teach us to breathe into impermanence—to find steadiness not by clinging, but by letting go.

2. Scripture

Sacred texts are not mere historical documents; they are luminous pathways into the human soul. Whether reading the Bible, Bhagavad Gita, Qur'an, Tao Te Ching, or Buddhist sutras, scripture invites contemplation more than instruction. Read slowly. Read prayerfully. Let the words speak beyond the intellect—into the heart's knowing.

> *"Don't be afraid, for I am with you."*—Isaiah 41:10
> *"Do not worry about tomorrow..."*—Matthew 6:34
> *"They will have no fear, nor will they grieve."*—Qur'an, 2:38
> *"Perform your duty... abandoning all attachment to success or failure."*—Bhagavad Gita

Each of these voices from diverse traditions speaks of a God who meets us in the moment—not in certainty, but in trust.

3. Rituals of Remembrance

Rituals are sacred choreography for the soul—grounding us in the eternal through the rhythms of daily life. Lighting a candle, walking a labyrinth, receiving communion, keeping the Sabbath—these gestures tether us to the holy.

Theologian Eric Carter notes that Sabbath observance can reduce stress and anxiety while enhancing wellbeing. Whether kneeling for the Eucharist or pausing for sunset prayer, rituals invite presence, peace, and participation in the sacred.

4. Prayer

Prayer is not always words. Sometimes it is silence. Sometimes it is the ache of the heart or a single whispered name. It is the soul reaching out—and sometimes, receiving a whisper in return.

Even science honors its mystery. In a well-known study by Harris. et al. (1999), intercessory prayer was associated with improved outcomes for cardiac patients. While the mechanism remains hidden, the fruits are often unmistakable: peace, clarity, healing, and presence.

5. Five Breathing Practices

Breath is the bridge between body and spirit—always present, always faithful. Intentional breathing calms the nervous system, quiets the mind, and returns us to the present moment. A few practices include:

- **Abdominal Breathing**: Expanding the belly, not just the chest, to soothe the stress response by stimulating the parasympathetic vagus nerve to "rest and digest".
- **Slow Breathing**: Six counts in, six counts out—slows the tempo of body and mind.
- **4-7-8 Breathing**: Inhale 4 – Hold 7 – Exhale 8. Deeply calming and restorative.
- **Pursed-Lip Breathing**: Slow exhalation through pursed lips—a soft release.
- **Box Breathing**: Inhale 4 – Hold 4 – Exhale 4 – Hold 4. A rhythm of reset.

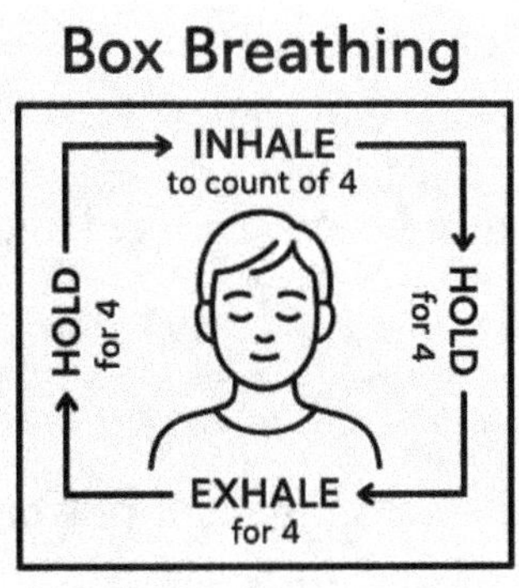

Box breathing

When breathing is practiced with mindfulness, it becomes prayer-in-motion.

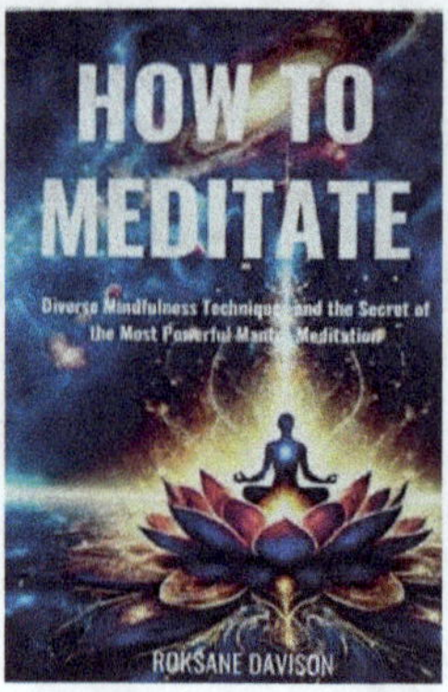

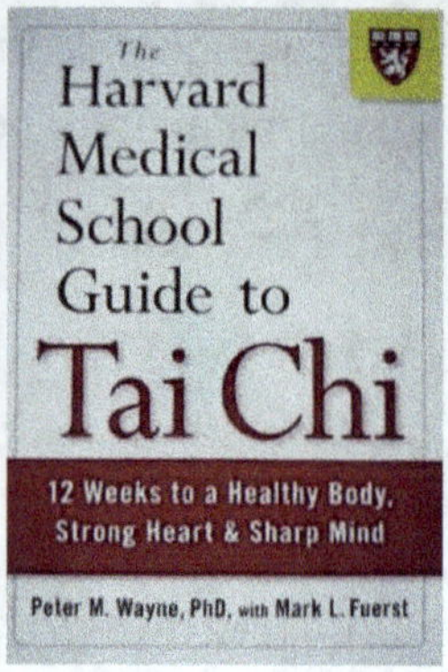

6. Meditation and Contemplation

Meditation and contemplation anchor us in the now. They are the art of resting in being—without fixing, solving, or striving. These practices teach us to witness our thoughts and environment without judgment and to open to the stillness beneath them.

Benefits include:

- Presence in the now
- Calm amid anxiety
- Acceptance of not-knowing
- Self-compassion and clarity
- Deepened spiritual connection

In contemplation, silence becomes sacred and uncertainty becomes communion.

7. Yoga and Tai Chi

These ancient practices offer embodied prayer—uniting movement, breath, and stillness.

Yoga links breath with posture, creating spaciousness in both body and spirit. It cultivates self-compassion and present-moment awareness.

Tai Chi flows in meditative motion, harmonizing the nervous system and building emotional balance.

Through these practices, the body becomes a sacred vessel—not to escape, but to inhabit fully.

8. Walking

Walking can be in one's neighborhood, and should be done mindfully, that is, observing trees, flowing plants, streams, the sky, and the people you may encounter—greeting briefly with a smile. Following the walk, journaling the experience can be insightful. A walk can also be in nature, at a park, or on a beach.

9. Labyrinth Slow Walk

Many have been blessed to discover a nearby Labyrinth (pictured at end of this chapter) and involves walking the labyrinth path slowly, thoughtfully, mindfully, and prayerfully. This has been an ancient practice and can be done alone or with a group led by a religious leader who blesses the walk.

10. Retreats

Retreats offer sacred pause. Whether in a monastery, cabin, or woodland trail, retreats allow time for quiet, reflection, and communion. They remind us that sacred ground is often found when we step away from noise of everyday life. Religious retreat centers offer spiritual direction, mindfulness training, and space for grief or healing. The retreat may end, but the inner spaciousness often lingers.

11. Nature

Creation itself is a form of scripture. Wind, stone, trees, stars—all bear the fingerprints of the divine. To walk in nature is to walk in a living cathedral. Let nature's quiet majesty speak to your soul.

"Adopt the pace of nature. Her secret is patience."—Ralph Waldo Emerson

"The poetry of the earth is never dead."—John Keats

12. Mystical Experiences

Mystical moments—flashes of unity, peace, or divine nearness—often arrive unbidden. We cannot force them, but we can cultivate receptivity. Stillness, prayer, awe, and grief all create the conditions in which mystery may touch us.

The Dalai Lama teaches that inner peace, born of meditation and compassion, is the wellspring of a meaningful life—especially in times of uncertainty.

13. Personal Narratives

Every life is a sacred story. The valleys, the mountaintops, the awakenings and doubts—all become part of the soul's unfolding. In bereavement groups I've facilitated, stories of loss have become vessels of healing. They share love and carry grace.

To speak honestly—and to listen deeply—is itself a spiritual practice.

14. Legacy

Spiritual practice shapes not only who we are, but what we leave behind. Our legacy is not only in accomplishments, but in how we forgive, serve, and love.

In families, legacies of courage and kindness become touchstones for generations. When we live with compassion, we plant seeds that bloom long after we're gone.

15. Community

We are not meant to walk through mystery alone. Spiritual friendships, faith communities, circles of trust—these are sanctuaries of belonging. In shared prayer or silence, questions or laughter, we remember we are not alone.

Together, we carry one another through the fog—each voice a candle in the dark.

16. Personal Journey

There is no map for the soul's path. Each of us walks a unique way. To honor your unfolding, even in uncertainty, is a sacred act.

Be kind to yourself. Trust the quiet guidance within—the nudges, the dreams, the synchronicities. The path is forming, even when hidden.

17. Literature

Many respected authors have written on the topics I have mentioned above. Many book covers are depicted in this book to show what is available. Avail yourself and you will be blessed.

A Practice of Grace

All these practices—from breath to silence, from community to solitude—are bound by one thread: grace. The spiritual life is not about perfection, but presence. There will be confusion, loss, and doubt. When that happens, return to the breath. Return to love. Return to what is simple and true. Let yourself be held—by God, by others, by the mystery that pulses at the heart of life.

Concluding Comments

In this second part of our journey, we have explored the nature of **Mystery**—in belief, in God, in creation, and in the sacred rhythms that sustain us. We have found that mystery is not the absence of meaning, but the presence of something deeper than comprehension. And we have learned to meet it not with fear, but with reverence.

Now, we prepare to step into the third part of this journey: **Miracles**.

Are miracles rare exceptions to natural law, or are they signs of a greater reality always at work—just beneath the surface? What happens when mystery breaks through the ordinary, revealing glimpses of divine intention and intervention? In the next chapter, we explore the nature of miracles—through science, story, and sacred experience. We ask not only *"Do miracles happen?"* but *"What do they mean?"*

Let us walk forward—eyes open, hearts expectant—into **Part III: Miracles**. But first, one question to consider, then look at the **labyrinth** pictured below:

- *Which of the spiritual practices in this chapter have you found to be a blessing or wish to explore?*

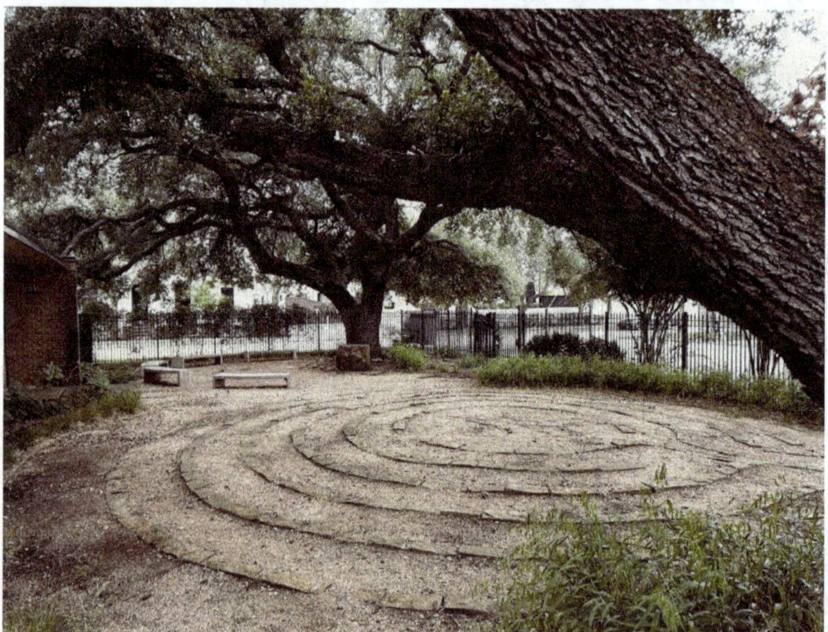

Labyrinth at Grace Episcopal Church, Houston
Picture taken by Fr. John K Graham

PART III: MIRACLES

Introduction to Part III: Miracles

Years ago, a woman in hospice care lay quietly, her breathing shallow, her family gathered in vigil. She had not spoken in days, and the doctors said she might not last the night. Then, just as the sun set, she opened her eyes, smiled broadly, and spoke the name of her late husband—gone for more than a decade. "He's here," she whispered. A moment later, she exhaled her final breath, peaceful, radiant. The room was silent yet charged with a presence no one could name.

Was this a miracle?

The story is not unusual. Healthcare workers, chaplains, and family members often share moments like this—events that defy easy explanation, that touch something deep within us, and stir a sense of mystery. We can explain away the science: final bursts of neural activity, cultural scripts, or hallucinations. But these explanations often feel incomplete. As if the language of biology cannot quite capture the fullness of what occurred.

In our modern age—shaped by science, skepticism, and the search for proof—the very word "miracle" can trigger resistance. Are we really to believe that the laws of physics can be suspended? That divine intervention overrides natural order? Since the Enlightenment, thinkers like David Hume have framed miracles as violations of natural law—improbable, unprovable, and therefore, for many, unacceptable.

And yet, the mystery remains. Something unexpected happens. Healing occurs against all odds. Timing becomes uncanny. Nature astonishes. Hearts open. And lives change.

Why Miracles Matter

This section of the book, Miracles, is not an argument to convince the skeptic or a catalog of supernatural claims. Instead, it's an invitation: to reexamine what we mean by "miracle," to explore the scriptural and philosophical traditions that have shaped our understanding, and to consider how we might experience the miraculous—not necessarily by breaking natural law, but by revealing deeper truths within it.

We'll explore:

- How miracles were defined historically and the impact of Enlightenment thought
- What the Bible actually says about miracles, signs, and wonders
- Modern perspectives that allow room for both science and awe
- Stories that challenge assumptions and inspire reflection

We'll also consider this: perhaps the greatest miracle is not something that suspends the laws of nature—but something that awakens us to the beauty, mystery, and meaning already present in the world.

After this poem, we will begin by exploring what exactly we mean by "miracle."

On Pain

And a woman spoke, saying, Tell us of Pain.
And he said:
Your pain is the breaking of the shell that encloses your understanding.
Even as the stone of the fruit must break, that its heart may stand in the sun, so must you know pain.
And could you keep your heart in wonder at the daily miracles of your life your pain would not seem less wondrous than your joy;
And you would accept the seasons of your heart, even as you have always accepted the seasons that pass over your fields.
And you would watch with serenity through the winters of your grief.

Much of your pain is self-chosen.
It is the bitter potion by which the physician within you heals your sick self.
Therefore, trust the physician, and drink his remedy in silence and tranquility:
For his hand, though heavy and hard, is guided by the tender hand of the Unseen,
And the cup he brings, though it burn your lips, has been fashioned of the clay which the Potter has moistened with His own sacred tears.

Poem by Kahlil Gibran (1883-1931)
Public domain, Wikimedia Commons

Chapter 13—Miracles Defined

Re-defining the Remarkable

When we hear the word miracle, many of us think of something dramatic—a blind man who suddenly sees, a storm that stops on command, or a terminal illness inexplicably cured. For centuries, miracles have been portrayed as divine disruptions, violations of the natural order that point unmistakably to the hand of God. But is that really what a miracle is?

In our time, shaped by science and reason, this traditional definition has become increasingly difficult for many to accept. Skeptics often argue, "If a miracle means breaking the laws of physics, then they cannot happen." The challenge isn't only disbelief; it's the definition itself. After two compelling stories we will look at a more acceptable definition of miracles.

Two Compelling Stories

Michael Egnor, M.D. is a neurosurgeon, who has shared his miraculous story in a book entitled, *The Immortal Mind: A Neurosurgeon's Case for the Existence of the Soul* (Egnor & O'Leary, 2025). After medical school and completing a residency in Neurosurgery, everything was going well for Michael and his wife, especially when they were blessed with a beautiful baby boy they loved instantly. Months passed with their son developing normally until they began to notice their son wasn't smiling or making eye contact with them. Being a physician who cared for patients with brain and mental problems, this terrified Michael who felt certain their son had autism. He began having nightmares and imagined his son growing up but being unable to know or love them. Time passed with no improvement in his son's condition which caused him to become even more anxious for his son's wellbeing.

One day, Dr. Egnor received a call to see a patient in a Catholic hospital in a nearby town. After seeing his patient, as Michael was leaving he happened to walk pass the hospital's chapel and said, "I don't believe in God, but I'll do anything now. I just want my son to know me." He went into the chapel, knelt, and said, "God, I don't know if you exist, but I need help. I am terrified that my son is autistic. It's agony to have a child who will never know or love me."

Instantly, Michael heard a voice in his head that he knew was not his own. This was something he had never experienced, and the voice answered his prayer saying, "But that's what you are doing to me. You don't look at me or talk to me either." Michael collapsed on the floor before the altar. He only heard a few words but knew he had heard God and realized God knew him intimately, had been watching him with love and wisdom all his life, and that God knew him even better than he knew himself. Michael prayed, "Lord, I won't be autistic with you any longer. Please heal my son, and please heal me." When Michael arose from the chapel floor, no longer an atheist. For the first time in his life neurosurgeon Dr. Michael Egnor knew God was real and he was transformed, a new man. In his book, Michael has written:

> A few days after my prayer in the chapel, I went home in the evening to my son's six-month birthday celebration. That night, he was behaving like a completely normal child, looking us in the eye, smiling and laughing. I knew I had experienced a miracle. It seemed as if, just as I had stopped ignoring the Lord, He had also allowed my son to see me. The following Easter, I was baptized, along with my son and other members of my family (Egnor & O'Leary, 2025).

Now that I have shared this story I am concerned that parents with a child who has autism will be distressed because their prayers have not been heard. Why this happens is a mystery and a heart-breaking one. Some will say Michael's child wasn't autistic and it was just a coincidence that his son responded after Michael's experience in the Catholic chapel. That is a plausible explanation, but Dr. Egnor believes he heard God speak to him and that he experienced a miracle.

One more thing I wish to say. Who can say that a child who has autism cannot communicate love for his or her parents? I am fairly certain parents with autistic children can share their unique story of connecting with their autistic child and feeling their connection, too.

Another remarkable story of healing. Professor of Clinical Pediatrics at Stritch School of Medicine at Loyola University, Chicago, Eugene Diamond, M.D. (2008) shared this story in an article entitled, "Miracles." In 1976, an eleven-year-old girl named Cirolli D. was brought to the orthopedic clinic at the University Hospital in Catania, Sicily. She had developed a painful swelling in her right knee. A biopsy confirmed every parent's worst fear: Ewing's sarcoma, an aggressive and often deadly bone cancer. The physicians recommended immediate amputation of the leg followed by radiation therapy. Her parents, overwhelmed and distraught, declined the treatment and returned home. Back in Palermo, a remarkable wave of compassion arose. Schoolchildren began collecting money to send Cirolli to Lourdes, the famed site of Marian apparitions and reported healings. Her pilgrimage took place from August 5–13, 1976.

What happened next was not immediate or dramatic—but it was steady and mysterious. By December of that same year, her symptoms began to resolve. Follow-up x-rays showed no evidence of the tumor that once threatened her life. The healing continued to hold. Cirolli's family returned to Lourdes in 1977 and reported the apparent disappearance of the cancer to the Medical Bureau. The case was thoroughly investigated over the next three years, with biopsy slides and imaging reviewed by independent experts. No recurrence was found. Ultimately, her cure was declared "scientifically inexplicable" and presented to the International Medical Committee of Lourdes, where it was considered as a possible miracle (Diamond, 2008). Stories like eleven-year-old Cirolli's remind us that the boundary between the ordinary and the extraordinary is not always as clear as we might assume. To some, her healing is a sign—a glimpse of divine presence breaking into human life. To others, it remains a mystery yet to be explained.

Throughout history, the idea of miracles has carried different meanings, shaped by theology, philosophy, and the evolution of science. Before we can explore modern interpretations, it's worth revisiting how miracles have been defined in the past—and how those definitions continue to influence the way we perceive them today.

A Historical Definition—Its Limits

Much of the modern skepticism surrounding miracles can be traced back to the 18th century Scottish philosopher David Hume. He argued that a miracle is "a violation of the laws of nature" and that such a claim should always be met with suspicion unless the evidence is overwhelming. This view dominated Enlightenment thinking and has since shaped much of the Western world's understanding of miracles.

But this definition was never the only one.

As early as 1755, Pope Benedict XIV offered a more nuanced view: **"A miracle is an event that exceeds the power of visible and corporeal nature only."** In other words, what is termed a miracle may not violate the natural laws of physics. Pope Benedict XIV also emphasized that a miracle must be of religious significance—its meaning matters as much as its mechanics.

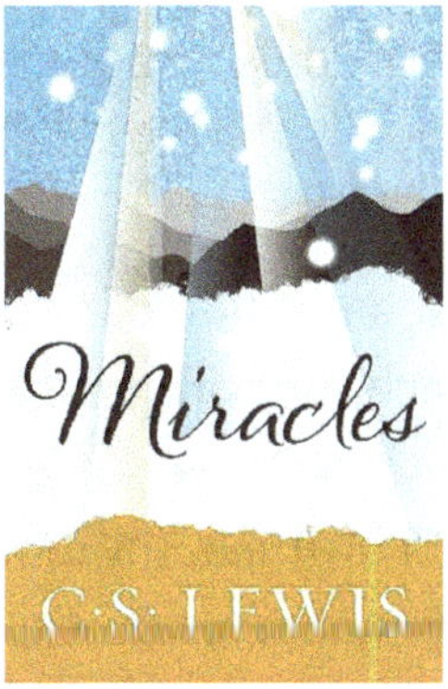

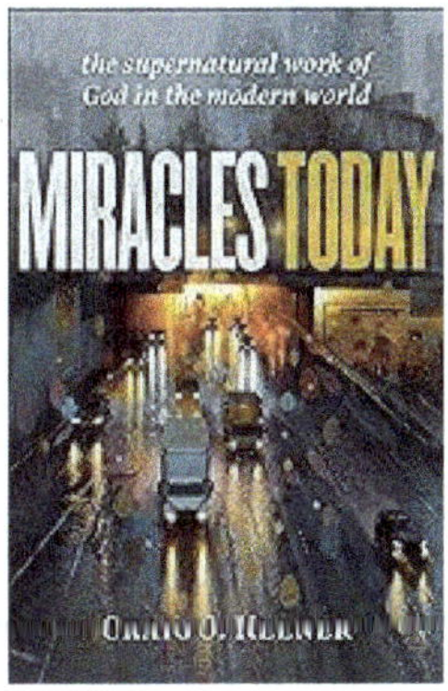

Writing in the mid-20th century, C. S. Lewis (1947) expanded on this idea. In his thoughtful book entitled *Miracles*, he argued that miracles do not cancel nature but rather *appear* in a way that is consistent with God's purposes. A miracle, in Lewis's view, is not a contradiction of natural law, but a divine act that enters the system from beyond it. Like a conductor stepping onto the stage is intentional to unite multiple instruments and create music, not chaos.

Biblical Perspectives: Signs and Wonders

Interestingly, the Bible itself does not define miracles as law-breaking events. The most common Hebrew word for miracle, *oth* (אוֹת) means a "sign." In Genesis 4:15 God placed a sign on Cain lest someone try to kill him. In this case, *oth* pointed beyond itself to God, like a road sign that doesn't exist for its own sake, but to direct us somewhere else. In Greek, the New Testament uses the word *semeion*, also meaning sign, and teras, which translates as "wonder."

This tells us something important: biblical miracles were not primarily about spectacle. They were symbolic acts that revealed something about **the nature of God**—his compassion, his love, his justice, or His Presence. When Jesus healed the sick, multiplied food, or calmed storms, the point was not to show off divine power, but to point people toward deeper spiritual truths. These signs invited belief, evoked wonder, and stirred the hearts of those who witnessed them.

Toward a Modern Understanding

Given all this, perhaps we need a new definition of miracles for today. Not one that pits faith against science, but one that welcomes both wonder and understanding.

What if a miracle is not the violation of natural law, but rather the appearance of divine meaning within natural events?

What if a miracle is best understood as an event that evokes awe, transforms lives, and opens the heart to something greater than itself?

This **reframing** allows us to see miracles not only in stories from long ago, but in our own lives—when an addiction is broken, when reconciliation seems impossible and yet happens, when grief gives way to peace, when hope unexpectedly returns.

Physicians' View of Religion & Spirituality on Health

Farr Curlin et al. (2007) surveyed 2000 practicing US physicians to estimate their observations as to how patients mention Religion and Spirituality (R/S) issues on health and how R/S influences health. The authors state, "few topics in medicine generate more disagreement than the relationship between religion and health." For this reason, the opinion of physicians as to what they observed in the practice of medicine with their patients was felt to be important.

The survey revealed most physicians (56%) believed that R/S had much or very much influence on heath, but few (6%) believed that R/S often changed "hard" medical outcomes. Most physicians (76%) felt R/S often helps patients cope, gives patients a positive state of mind (75%), and that patients receive emotional and practical support from their religious community. Most physicians (82%) believe that R/S positively impacts health.

The survey also sought to determine whether the religious beliefs of the physician may affect the interaction with patients concerning R/S issues. Protestant physicians were more likely to report that their patients bring up R/S issues and are more likely to believe that God intervenes in a patient's health, that R/S helps them to cope, and that R/S helps prevent "hard" medical outcomes. Catholics were more likely to believe that God intervenes and that R/S helps patients to cope. They are less likely to believe that R/S causes negative emotions. Physicians of other religions were more likely to report their patients bring up R/S issues, that God intervenes, and that R/S strongly influences health and can prevent hard medical outcomes. And physicians from the Southern US states were more likely to report their patients often mention R/S issues. Physicians in the West and Northeast were less likely to believe that R/S influences health in strong and positive ways. Nevertheless, most physicians believe that R/S has a substantial and generally positive influence on patients' health and that "on occasion" the influence is due to divine intervention.

The survey indicates that from the perspective of the physicians surveyed, overt miracles are not commonly witnessed in their practice of medicine. Nevertheless, most physicians were able to say that religious and spirituality practices are a positive influence on their patients and that "on occasion" the positive influence may be due to divine intervention.

The Greatest Miracle of All? Life Itself

If we zoom out far enough, we come upon what might be the greatest miracle of all: the fact that we are here, alive and well on planet Earth. We have approached this previously when considering the mystery of life.

Modern science has revealed a universe so "finely tuned" for life that even the smallest changes in its fundamental forces would have rendered life impossible.

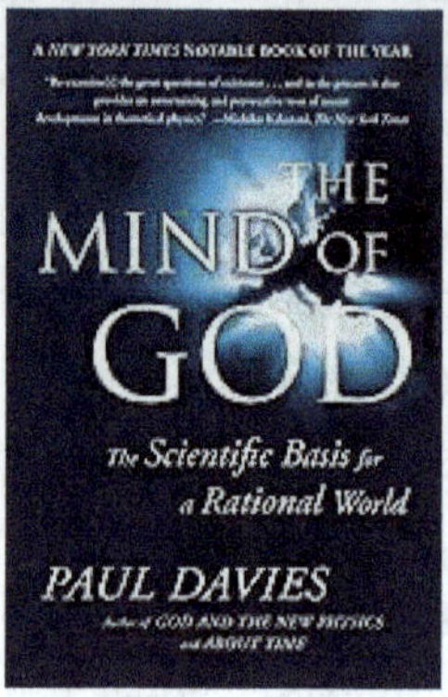

In his book *The Mind of God*, physicist Paul Davies writes, "There is now broad agreement among physicists and cosmologists that the Universe is in several respects 'fine-tuned' for life."

As early as 1961, physicist Robert H. Dicke pointed out that certain forces—like gravity and electromagnetism—had to be calibrated with breathtaking precision for life to arise. Even Stephen Hawking, who did not profess belief in a personal God, acknowledged the wonder: "The values of these numbers seem to have been very finely adjusted to make possible the development of life."

Is this fine-tuning simply random luck? A cosmic accident? Or is it a sign—an *oth*, a *semeion*—that something beyond us is at work?

Concluding Comments: Opening to Wonder

In the end, perhaps a miracle is not something that suspends reality, but something that awakens us to its depth. Not something that breaks the laws of nature, but something that reveals the heart of the One who wrote them.

In the chapters that follow, we'll look at stories—ancient and modern—that illustrate this broader vision of the miraculous. We'll consider the role of healing, timing, transformation, and even suffering, in revealing the presence of the sacred.

And we'll ask, with open hearts and curious minds: what if the miraculous is not rare at all, but hidden in plain sight? Join me in the next chapter where we look at the Miracle of Life.

Questions for further thought and consideration:

- *In this chapter two stories were presented that were said to be evidence of miracles (Dr. Egnor and an eleven-year-old girl who was taken to the Lourdes). What are your thoughts about miracles? Have you or someone you loved experienced a miracle?*
- *Not all prayers for a miracle are granted. Does this mean "miracles" are just coincidences?*
- *If someone prays for a miracle and it is not granted, how could this affect one's faith?*
- *What do you think about the statement that the greatest miracle of all is life itself?*

Chapter 14—The Miracle of Life and the Fine-Tuned Universe

If miracles are signs that stir wonder, then perhaps the most awe-inspiring sign of all is the fact that we exist—that life, in all its fragile complexity, has emerged in a universe that appears precisely "tuned" to allow for it. The farther we explore the cosmos, and the deeper we delve into the nature of matter, the more astonishing this truth becomes.

What is Life?

Living things can be differentiated from non-life in many ways. The living has the innate ability to sustain itself, adapt, and reproduce, properties that non-living lack. Living things are also composed of cells that grow and change throughout their lifetime. Cells require nutrients for energy and a secure, a life-friendly environment for their survival. Eventually, the living die (perhaps not Immortal Jellyfish and Planaria). Finally, living things are not inert or static—life expresses itself by organizing and cooperating with other living things to their benefit, while not always for the well-being of our planet and other creatures. Living beings positively or negative impact other life forms and the planet itself.

The Cell—Building Block of Life

For most of my life I have been amazed as I learn more about our vast and awe-inspiring Universe, and lately I have been equally amazed as I learn more about the very small, carbon-based cells that are the basis for life on our planet. Each plant or animal cell consists of hundreds of trillions of atoms (yes, trillions) yet is only a millionth the size of a grain of sand (yes, a millionth). Though very small, each cell has a remarkable architecture within a multilayered outer cell wall which "knows" when to admit nutrients and when to reject that which would be harmful.

In his book, *The Amazing Cell*, biochemist Michael Denton (2020) writes:

> The unique fitness of the cell to serve as the fundamental unit of life is manifest by its amazing abilities and the diversity of functions it performs.

For example, within each cell there is a complex internal structure with a central Nucleus bathed in cytoplasm containing organelles—Mitochondria, Golgi complex, an Endoplasmic Reticulum, Microtubules, Lysosomes, Ribosomes, and Vacuoles. Each structure has a specific role constantly working to carry out essential life processes within the cell.

As to the diversity of functions, the Nucleus contains the cell's DNA with informational instructions for all cellular activities. DNA's structure is amazing—the building blocks are nucleotides consisting of sugar and phosphate groups with four nitrogenous bases—adenine (A), thymine (T), guanine (G), and cytosine (C), positioned on a double-helix of two DNA strands that run in opposite directions such that Adenine is always paired with thymine, and guanine is always paired with cytosine. Can we really see DNA as an accident of nature?

Mitochondria are the "powerhouse" of the cell, converting nutrients into usable energy for cellular function. The Endoplasmic Reticulum is involved in protein and lipid synthesis. The Golgi Apparatus processes proteins and other molecules for transport within the cell or transport outside. Lysosomes have enzymes that break down waste materials and cellular debris.

When contained within the body of an animal or plant, cells are joined to become an interconnecting and intercommunicating community such that the sum of the parts is greater than that of any single cell. Cells communicate with each other through signaling molecules and receptors on the surface of the cell. The growth of cells occurs through cell division and differentiation. Clearly, cells are a highly organized, complex system where intercellular processes work together to maintain life and carry out specific functions within the body.

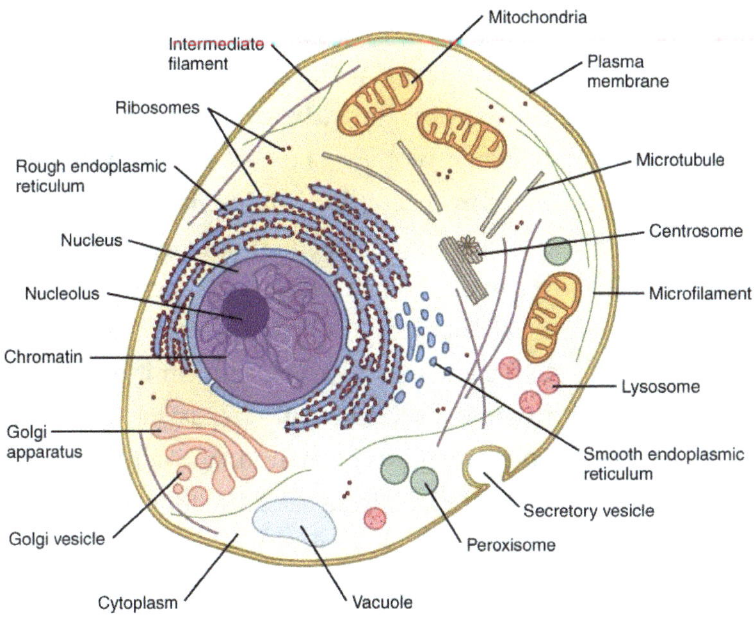

Public Domain Source: Creative Commons, OpenStax via Wikimedia Commons, licensed under CC-BY 4.0.

The Cell and Artificial Intelligence (AI)

With the progress of artificial intelligence (AI) the complex design and function of biological cells began to be used as a metaphor for machine learning, and vice versa. In an interesting article, computer scientists, Bongard and Levin (2021) write:

> Living things are amazing—they show resilience, purposeful action, unexpected complexity. The have true "skin in the game"—they actively care about what happens and can be rewarded or punished by experience. They surprise us at every turn by their ingenuity, their wholism, and their resistance to naïve reductionist approaches to analysis and control.

That being true, Bongard and Levin (2021) say it is time to realize that the technological advancements of artificial intelligence has reached a level of **human-AI hybridization** that is erasing the classical boundaries between biology and intelligent machines. For example, machines are now becoming highly integrated with the living for sensory augmentation, cochlear implants, brain-machine interfaces, brain implants, enhancement of performance, the implantation of internal devices to control the rate of heart contractions and to deliver insulin and neurotransmitters. Machines may soon read memories and insert new ones bypassing the biological mechanisms of perception, memory formation, and communication.

Bongard and Levin conclude: "Today the function, cognition and status of these hybrid systems make it clear no simple dichotomy can be drawn between life and machine." This is a profound statement which introduces the subject of what is the meaning of life—a subject worthy of thoughtful consideration later in this book.

The Meaning of Life

Laying aside the issue raised by artificial intelligence, the mystery of the origin of life has long fostered heated and passionate controversy that affects our understanding of the ultimate meaning of human life. On the one hand, there are those who affirm a supranatural explanation and believe that at creation human life was formed in God's image. Others believe aliens have visited and brought life to Earth, and scientists continue to search for an explanation that fits within their materialist paradigm.

For example, theoretical physicist Paul Davies (2000) has proposed that life may not have originated on Earth; instead, life may have been deposited here from outer space. In the early formative years of our planet, meteorites, comets, and asteroids have penetrated Earth's dense, hot atmosphere and plunged into land and oceans superheated by volcanic eruptions, possibly bringing bio forms with each impact. This means, life may have begun deep within the Earth's crust or in the depth of our oceans (Parker et al., 2014). Others have responded by saying the very superheated environment of early Earth may have been incompatible with life. This was a reasonable assumption until plants and fish were found surviving quite well in the deepest trenches of the Pacific ocean, where it was thought life was impossible.

Yet, believing life was deposited on our planet by meteorites or aliens merely displaces the origin of life from Earth to outer space. The question remained how did life begin there? To answer that question, in the early 1950s a series of scientific experiments began in chemical laboratories that have convinced most scientists to believe that we have an understanding as to how life could have begun on structures in outer space where atmospheric conditions may have been more conducive to organic synthesis than on Earth.

The Miller-Urey Experiment: A Glimpse into the Origins of Life

In 1953, a University of Chicago graduate student named Stanley L. Miller, under the guidance of Nobel laureate, Harold Clayton Urey, began to explore in a chemical laboratory one of humanity's most profound questions: *How did life begin on Earth?* Considered by many today to be the greatest discovery in biology of the 20th century, their experiment became the foundation of origin-of-life research, bridging chemistry with the spiritual awe of creation.

Miller and Urey were inspired by the idea proposed decades earlier by Alexander Oparin and J. B. S. Haldane—scientists who, independently, envisioned early Earth as a kind of "primordial soup." They imagined oceans filled with simple organic compounds that were being stirred by electrical energy (lightning) slowly evolving toward the complexity of life. But it wasn't until Miller-Urey's laboratory experiment that this idea gained broad scientific attention.

Simulating Primitive Earth Atmosphere

To recreate an early Earth environment, Miller and Urey designed a closed glass apparatus that mimicked the conditions of the young planet's atmosphere. Into the system the following was introduced to duplicate the primitive atmosphere of the earth:

- Water vapor (to simulate ancient oceans),
- Methane (CH_4), Ammonia (NH_3), and Hydrogen (H_2)—gases thought to be present in the early Earth atmosphere—were circulated past an electric discharge to simulate lightning, an abundant energy source in the early planet's atmosphere.

What They Found

On the first day water in the flask turned pink. After one week, the contents of the water flask were a murky reddish-brown. Also, yellow organic compounds were found absorbed on silica. Because the water was boiling, Miller felt contamination by living organisms was not present. A paper chromatogram chemical analysis revealed the spontaneous formation of several amino acids—glycine and both alpha- and beta- alanine. Other amino acids were thought to be present in smaller amounts but not measured. The three amino acids identified are among the twenty building blocks of proteins required for organic life.

Consistent with traditional scientific caution when reporting research findings, Miller wrote, "In this apparatus an attempt was made to duplicate a primitive atmosphere of the earth, and not to obtain the optimum conditions for the formation of amino acids." He continued, "Although in this case the total yield was small for the energy expended, it is possible that, with more efficient apparatus this type of process would be a way of commercially producing amino acids."

The response was extraordinary. Miller had demonstrated, for the first time in a controlled setting, that organic molecules could be synthesized from inorganic gases under conditions that resemble the atmosphere of early Earth. Life, it appeared, could emerge from the laws of chemistry itself—given the proper environment, energy, and time.

Reflections and Implications

The Miller-Urey experiment has been repeated and refined many times since 1953, including an article published in the *Journal of Visualized Experiments* by Parker et al. (2014) that carefully explained a complex protocol required to conduct Miller-Urey Experiments. Their work used updated equipment to ensure safety and improve reproducibility, but the core insight remained: life's molecular precursors can arise in the absence of life—a finding that supports the possibility of life emerging elsewhere in the cosmos.

Yet, for all their scientific rigor, Miller-Urey experiments have not able to create atoms or molecules, much less a living cell. This has opened the door for some Christian conservatives to say that not being able to create life in the laboratory is proof of the biblical origin of life (Bergman, 2017). Which, of course, is not a scientifically valid assumption. Furthermore, the question remains as to what kind of universe would allow simple molecules, exposed to lightning and time, to evolve to the level of human consciousness? Might there be, as I explore in this book, a universal consciousness—a divine intelligence—that not only set the conditions for life but imbued it with purpose?

Considering quantum theory and the concept of an Information Universe, one could view Miller and Urey's work as a glimpse into the divine code of existence—where from randomness emerged form, from chaos came pattern, and from mere chemistry arose self-replicating life.

Whether the origin of life on our planet took place by an act of God, through visits by aliens, or by meteorite deposits in the depths of the Earth's oceans or crust, something remarkable took place 3.8 billion years ago that changed the destiny of Earth forever—organic life began for the first time on our planet. And at our birth, we entered our planet's long history and life has meaning because we are here.

Whether one sees this as the work of chance or the unfolding thought of God, the awe it inspires can surely be shared by scientist and mystic alike.

Scientists and the Fine-tuned Universe

Scientists have observed our universe appears to be "fine-tuned" for life. This suggests that the physical constants and laws of nature are not random but rather fall within extremely narrow ranges that make life—especially intelligent life—possible.

For example, if the gravitational constant were slightly weaker or stronger, stars might never have formed, or they would burn too quickly to host planets. If the strong nuclear force were even slightly different, atoms might never have held together. The balance is said to be so delicate that even the smallest deviation in one of many fundamental constants would render life as we know it impossible.

Some scientists describe this balance as a “cosmic hospitality”—a universe whose very fabric seems tailored for the emergence of sentient beings capable of wonder, creativity, and contemplation.

As mentioned in the last chapter, in his book, *The Mind of God* (1993), Paul Davies wrote: “There is now broad agreement among physicists and cosmologists that the Universe is in several respects ‘fine-tuned’ for life.”

Davies and others, including Robert H. Dicke and Freeman Dyson, have observed that our universe seems not only habitable but “improbably so.” Dicke proposed in 1961 that certain constants in nature must have been precisely calibrated, or life would not be possible anywhere.

Stephen Hawking, though not a theist, shared this sentiment in *A Brief History of Time* (1988):

> The laws of science... contain many fundamental numbers... The remarkable fact is that the values of these numbers seem to have been very finely adjusted to make possible the development of life.

Fine-tuning has led to two major schools of thought. Some interpret it as compelling evidence for an intelligent creator, one who designed the cosmos with purpose. Others suggest that we live in one of countless universes—**a Multiverse**—and that it’s not surprising that we find ourselves in the one universe that happens to allow life. After all, if it weren’t so, we wouldn’t be here to ask about the origin of life on our planet.

The debate continues, but what remains undeniable is that the universe is, at the very least, highly improbable and yet remarkably we are here.

The Miracle of Life: Fragility and Wonder

To repeat again, the reality of life on Earth can be seen as a miracle of improbability—yet human beings do exist and are alive and well on our tiny planet. For that reason alone, from the elegant design of a single cell to the staggering complexity of the human brain, every aspect of life testifies to something rare, something sacred.

Earth orbits a relatively stable star in a galactic neighborhood that is calm enough to allow evolution over billions of years. Our planet holds liquid water, a breathable atmosphere, and a magnetic field that shields us from solar radiation which the planet Mars does not have.

The conditions required for even microbial life are so exacting that scientists continue to debate whether life exists elsewhere in the universe at all. Despite our technological advances, we have not found factual evidence of life beyond Earth.

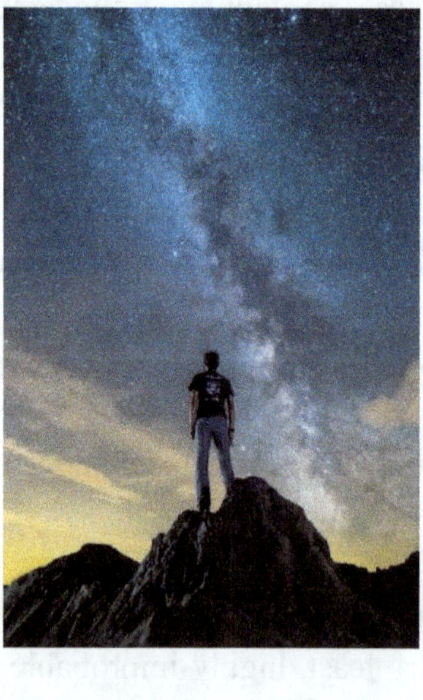

Gazing at Milky Way Stars at Pannecière lake, in Morvan National Park, France.
Photography by Benh LIEU SONG @flickr.com.
Public Domain licensed under the Creative Commons Attribution-Share Alike 4.0 International license. Wikimedia Commons.

Nevertheless, there are said to be over 200 billion stars in our Milky Way galaxy and billions—if not trillions—of galaxies are known to exist, surely many have planets in the "goldilocks range." This means it is perfectly logical to believe that life is just waiting to be discovered light-years away. But until then, we are left to marvel at the singular gift we know we possess: the miracle of life itself.

While no precise calculation can be given as to the probability of life having appeared on Earth, it does exist. And scientific evidence such as the Miller-Urey Experiments suggest it's not a totally improbable either. For this reason, understanding the exact mechanisms of life's origin remains a continuing focus for research.

Contemporary interfaith dialogue has increasingly recognized that while the metaphysical frameworks differ, the longing for divine intervention, healing, and hope is universally human. Miracles, East and West, function as sacred symbols—threshold moments when the veil between heaven and earth seems to lift, offering a glimpse of the eternal.

Concluding Comments

In this chapter we have journeyed from the intricate machinery of the living cell to the vast orchestration of the cosmos, from the frontiers of artificial intelligence to the timeless wonder of human consciousness. We have marveled at the fine-tuning of physical laws, pondered the mystery of our origins through the lens of both science and spirit, and glimpsed the sacred within the seemingly natural. Life, as we have seen, is not merely a biological phenomenon—it is a profound miracle woven into the very fabric of existence. And while the miracle of life offers a universal sign of wonder, it is through the lens of sacred literature that humanity has most often sought to understand, record, and respond to the miraculous.

In the next chapter, we will explore the impact of the "miracle" of artificial Intelligence (AI)—the opportunities and realistic concerns. I include this coming chapter because right now we can only anticipate the dramatic impact AI will have on our lives, yet it is important we begin that conversation and prepare our mind, heart, and spirit for what is ahead.

Before moving to the next chapter, it may be worthwhile to do personal reflection. Perhaps the following questions will help us reflect further on the underlying Miracle of Life.

- *When you consider the amazing fact we are alive today on this beautiful planet in the "goldilocks zone" with every provision for human life, against every improbability, what do you feel inside?*
- *We looked at the amazing complexity of a single organic cell. Bongard and Levin say: "Living things are amazing—they show resilience, purposeful action, unexpected complexity." What are your thoughts?*
- *Any thought about the Universe being fine-tuned?*
- *Hybridization is uniting biology and intelligent machines. Where can this benefit humanity? Any concerns?*

Chapter 15—The "Miracle" of Artificial Intelligence (AI)

While the rise of artificial intelligence (AI) does not meet the criteria of a divine miracle, what it has accomplished in its brief history borders on the miraculous—with even far greater possibilities unfolding. Most of us use AI every day without thinking twice, such as when we conduct a Google search. Yet the development of AI also raises serious questions we are only beginning to confront. But, first, let's look at the "Miracle" of AI.

A Glimpse at the "Miracle" of AI

In the course I took at Harvard on AI in Medicine, we learned the best way to view artificial intelligence (AI) is as a **partner** who assists in making certain tasks easier but not by replacing us, nor our wisdom, judgment, decision-making, or when considering humane and ethical matters. So, how can AI assist and be our partner in making life easier? As most of us have already discovered, AI is great at rapidly searching for information on internet search engines, and AI is good at recognizing grammatical and spelling errors when writing documents.

Processing data

AI also is extremely helpful in rapidly accomplishing large tasks. It can process information faster and more accurately than we humans. AI is also good at automating tasks and identifying insights that might otherwise be overlooked. This means it is wonderful in academic research projects involving large datasets, repetitive analysis, and pattern recognition. In particular, AI is excellent for accounting and finance and in creative arts—artistic paintings, writing, and music. Best of all, IA (Intelligence Amplification) may be able to make everyone appear to be a genius (super-intelligent). Imagine being the first one on the block or at work with IA, Intelligence Amplification.

Industrial Robots

Industry is rapidly making use of these skills with the use of robots. The value here is robots perform repetitive tasks 24-hours-a-day, 7-days-a-week without a vacation. They also engage in hazardous activities which have a high risk to human workers. They are good for tasks like welding, painting, assembly, handling of materials, boxing for delivery, and quality control. These tasks lead to increased efficiency, safety, and precision in manufacturing and agriculture.

Medical Care

It is anticipated that AI can assist a physician in making complex diagnoses and aid nursing by improving efficiency, safety of medication distribution, and with patient transport. Also, in time robots may provide companionship for long-term patients, addressing loneliness and promoting well-being. However, it would appear the presence of human doctors and caregivers will always remain essential.

AI-Enabled Physicians

In a recent issue of *JAMA*, two articles addressed the future of AI in healthcare. The press and social media have presented AI as better at diagnosis than a physician because AI did higher than average on medical exams. However, patient care involves much more than regurgitating facts. It involves the skill of reasoning and moral judgment that comes from years of one-on-one patient care. The doctor-patient relationship depends on communicating care, respect, empathy, and compassion—something only a human can truly give. Succi et al., (2025) addressed the opportunities and challenges to preparing future physicians so they become AI-augmented while ensuring that the quality of patient care remains at the highest level.

As I said earlier, AI works best as the physician's partner. This is the issue addressed in another *JAMA* article by Kenneth Mandl (2025) who describes how AI could reshape health care through direct-to-consumer (DTC) health care—that is, AI-to-patient care—without the oversight of a physician. Big Tech companies—Google, Open AI, Microsoft, and other firms have already begun gathering data and providing health care recommendations with chatbots. The question is how will these DTCs receive the oversight needed to ensure patient safety and privacy? At this time, it is not clear which governmental agency will be responsible, nor are guidelines in place. Another issue is whether the elderly and others will have difficulty accessing the technology. Availability of DTC's could result in greater inequities in the quality of healthcare received.

Robots in Healthcare

Robotic surgery has begun assisting the surgeon by enhancing precision and control, improving surgical outcomes. Typically, this means smaller incisions and less pain following the procedure. This became very personal for me when I developed cancer of the ascending colon. Instead of having major incisions and a colostomy, using robotics my surgeon was able to resect a third of my colon, and I went home the next day with little or no pain.

Post-operatively, robots can provide instruction to patients and families. If physical rehabilitation is required, robots can assist in the rehabilitation process and help patients regain their mobility and strength. In the future robots may be excellent in counseling one-on-one. Many people already admit to asking ChatGPT for advice instead of using a human counselor, and they appear to be pleased with the advice AI has shared.

Domestic Robots

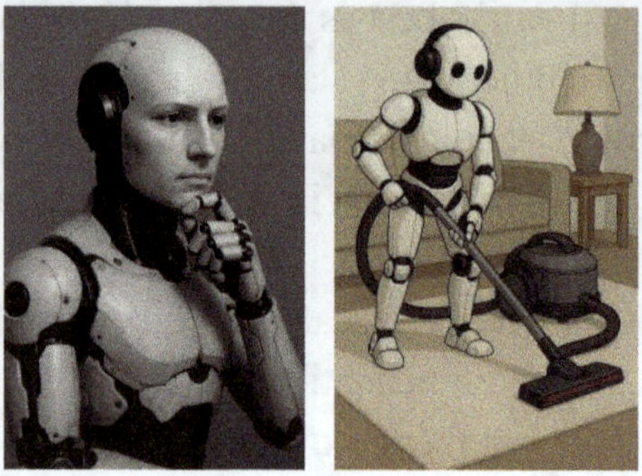

Robot on left ponders if it really wants to vacuum.

Soon, robots will be common in homes for chores, cleaning, lawn care, and companionship. This would be of great value for those who live alone and the elderly who need companionship, assistance with mobility, and with everyday tasks like getting dressed, taking baths, and preparing meals.

Automatic Cars

We already have automated cars on the road, including 18-wheeler trucks with no drivers. The impact will escalate when robotaxis become widely available. I have spoken to **visually-impaired** individuals who look forward to the day they can purchase an automated car, so they won't have to wait—sometimes for hours—for someone to pick them up. The freedom to jump into our car and head to our destination is something we often take for granted.

Concerns About AI

First, is the looming concern about loss of employment for countless people and the issue of inequality as to who will benefit—will the rich get richer while the rest of us are left without income or hope of future employment?

Loss of Employment

We are already aware the list of threatened jobs includes customer service and data entry clerks, accountants, receptionists, truck drivers, couriers, factory and warehouse workers, computer programmers, research analysts, paralegals, artists, and others too numerous to list. Yet, we are promised new jobs will be created, but the human element remains critical for many jobs as the following article makes clear.

Concern about AI Agents

Author, Mehul Gupta (2025, Jan 20), has worked with "AI Agents" since their inception and has posted an article on his website entitled "Why AI Agents will be a huge disaster."

Gupta begins by reminding us there have been many predictions that "2025 will be the year of Agents and that AI Agents will take over the world." He doesn't believe AI Agents will take over the world, but what is an AI Agent? I did an internet search, asking AI for the answer (Google search engine) and this is what I learned:

> An AI agent is a system or program that can autonomously perform tasks on behalf of a user or another system by designing its workflow and using available tools. They can range from simple question-answering to complex, multi-step tasks, and they can continuously learn and improve. AI agents are a type of AI that can perceive, learn, and interact with their environment in real-time (Google 2025, May 18).

This small glimpse of what AI Agents can do may raise the question as to why Gupta says this would be a "huge disaster?" Here are the reasons for his concern:

1. **The LLMs are still far from reaching 100% accuracy**. Gupta says because AI is not infallible, errors can have

significant consequences, especially in healthcare and the legal system. A human needs to be present to oversee choices before they are enacted.

2. **AI Agents have a hard time choosing tools**. Gupta points out AI often will rely on one tool where multiple tools may be needed, making AI Agent choices less reliable than a human worker who is familiar with which tools are best in which situation.
3. **Trust issues will always exist**. Trust is fundamental to any human-AI collaboration, and with every AI mistake, trust is eroded. The same is true for any area of human life or when financial matters are involved. People are cautious when making critical decisions.
4. **A human layer is still essential**. AI is excellent in repetitive, time-consuming tasks yet a human is needed to make judgment calls. AI lacks human empathy, intuition, and the ability to navigate moral complexities that arise every day in the real world.
5. **Biases exist and will persist in AI systems**. AI Agents' perform with data they are trained on. If the data has bias, it will be incorporated in AI's work. In the future, AI software may be programed to recognize biases and programmers can be alerted when a bias is found.
6. **Ethical and legal concerns**: AI Agents could open pandora's box. The question arises, who is responsible when an AI Agent makes a mistake? And who is accountable if an AI system is used for malevolent purposes or to commit fraud?
7. **Over-reliance on AI can lead to a loss of critical skills**. The fact is, the more we rely on AI Agents, the more certain it is we will lose our own problem-solving and critical-thinking abilities. Basically, over-dependence on AI will rob

human cognitive and reasoning capabilities, as well as losing essential skills over time.

Gupta says for these seven reasons governments, corporations, and tech companies need to establish clear guidelines and regulations to govern the use of AI Agents. Unchecked use of these systems could lead to untold harm to individuals including privacy violations and monopolies. Especially, when AI Agents are allowed to operate without human oversight.

More recently, many have raised the alarm that AI will soon become vastly more intelligent than human beings and could easily determine that human beings are a hinderance needing to be exterminated. Some feel it is naive to not realize this is a genuine concern that must be addressed before it takes place; afterwards will be too late.

A Final Thought

We are already adjusting to the presence of robots in the workplace, the marketplace, and in our homes. They will continue to shape our lives, often for the better—but sometimes at great social cost and growing socioeconomic inequities—with devastating effects. AI may be able to help solve these issues. Above all, we meet the opportunities and challenges of AI with hope. Humanity has repeatedly adapted and thrived amid great change. With our God-given creative insight and the wisdom of Universal Consciousness, may we navigate this new frontier with grace and purpose.

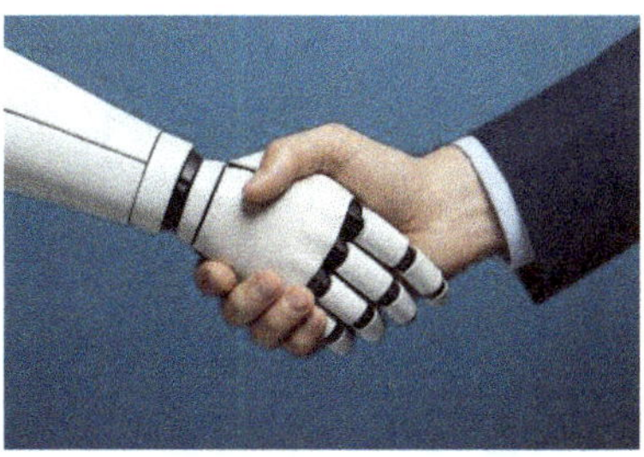

Are we ready to join hands with AI?

Concluding Comments

In the next chapter, we will look at how miracles have been revealed, interpreted, and cherished across the world's spiritual traditions—from the burning bush to walking on water, from sacred texts to oral traditions—as windows into the divine, affirming that the miraculous is not only real but deeply rooted in the stories that shape our souls.

Pondering about the future in an AI world invites us to think about the issues this chapter raised. You may find it helpful to reflect on these questions before moving to the next chapter.

- *When you think about all the possible benefits to AI, is there one that you or a loved one may find a blessing?*
- *Medical science has incorporated biotechnology in every generation—from the ECG to measure the rhythm of the heart, to fMRI studies of the brain, to the surgical insertion of prosthetic devices in hips and knees. What about incorporating AI in healthcare?*
- *Are you concerned about the possibility of people becoming unemployed due to AI? What remedies can you imagine in the suffering this will cause in people's lives? What role should governments play? What role can religious communities play?*
- *Any thoughts about Mehul Gupta's list of seven concerns he has for AI Agents? Do any one of the seven concerns particularly stand out to you? How can we keep a "human layer" in the loop? Are you concerned AI Agents may take over your job or that of a loved one?*
- *How can we address the concern that super-intelligent AIs will find humans a hinderance and are expendable?*

Chapter 16—Miracles in Sacred Literature

If the universe is miraculous, and life is miraculous, then the witness of world religions reveals another layer of divine activity—moments when the fabric of reality appears to shift, pointing beyond the natural order to the God who lovingly sustains it. Nowhere is this more vividly portrayed than in the pages of religious writings and scripture. The Bible, from beginning to end, is a story of miracles—signs and wonders that invite us to see the world not merely as it is, but as it can be when touched by divine presence.

Judaism: Divine Intervention in the Story of a People

The Hebrew Scriptures are filled with miraculous acts that reveal the power and purpose of God, especially as God relates to a chosen people. The very first words of Genesis set the tone for everything that follows: *"In the beginning, God created the heavens and the earth."* (Genesis 1:1) Creation itself is miraculous—the divine act of bringing order from chaos, light from darkness, and life from nothing.

The Old Testament records epic miracles that have shaped Jewish identity and continue to inspire wonder. God sends a great flood to cleanse the earth (Genesis 7–8) yet remembers Noah and offers a covenant marked by a rainbow. The ten plagues upon Egypt (Exodus 8–12) demonstrate divine justice and mercy, culminating in the dramatic parting of the Red Sea (Exodus 14), through which the Israelites escape bondage and head to the promised land.

The walls of Jericho fell, not by force, but by divine will and the faith-filled obedience of Joshua and the Israelites (Joshua 6). Below, in Daniel 3, the fiery furnace of Babylon, three faithful men emerge unscathed, because God met them in the flames.

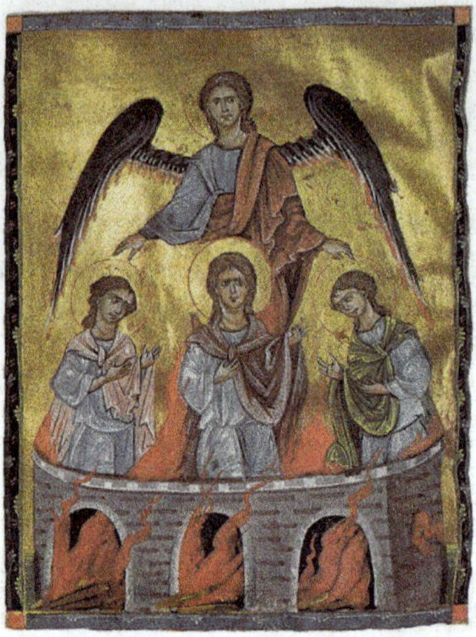

Three Men in Firey Furnace (1266) by Toros Roslin,
Public Domain, Wikimedia Commons. In1999, New York District Court ruled a photograph of the original requires no copyright protection.

These stories are more than historical claims; they are theological narratives, meant to reveal God's nature—God as deliverer, provider, protector, and sustainer. They are less about suspending natural law and more about revealing a deeper order: that God is not distant from creation but intimately involved in its unfolding.

New Testament Miracles: As Signs of the Kingdom

With the arrival of Jesus, miracles take on a new shape—personal, intimate, and deeply compassionate. His miracles are not displays of power for their own sake, but signs pointing to a greater reality: the inbreaking of God's kingdom.

The Gospels recount numerous miracles, from turning water into wine (John 2) to feeding thousands with a few loaves and fish

(Matthew 14, Mark 6, Luke 9, John 6). Jesus heals the sick, restores sight to the blind (Matthew 9), enables the lame to walk, and frees those tormented by unclean spirits. He walks on water, calms storms, and calls life out of death.

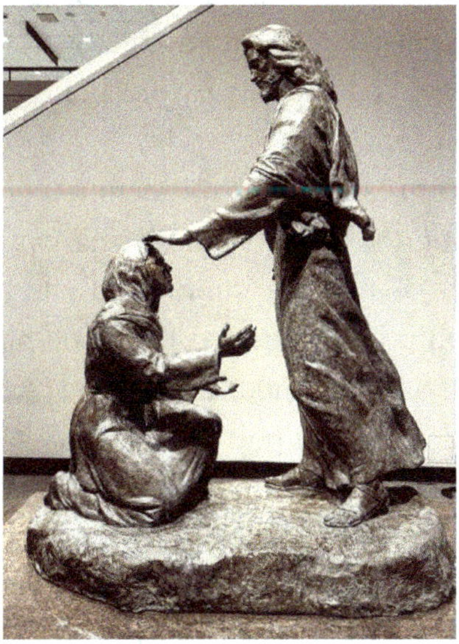

Jesus' Healing Touch statue, in lobby of Houston Methodist Hospital,
in Texas Medical Center, Houston
Photograph taken by Fr. John K Graham, Public domain

Perhaps most profoundly, Jesus raises Lazarus from the dead (John 11) and then, in the greatest miracle of all, in all four gospels, he rises from the grave (Matthew 28, Mark 16, Luke 24, John 20). The resurrection is not only a miracle—it is the cornerstone of Christian faith. It declares that love is stronger than death, and that God's power to heal and renew has no time limit.

Miracles in Jesus' ministry serve a dual purpose. They relieve suffering, yes—but they also reveal the nature of God. As signs, they point beyond themselves to a deeper truth: *"If you do not believe me, believe the works,"* Jesus said (John 10:38). They are not magic tricks or proof texts, but invitations to believe, to trust, and to follow.

Miracles in the Book of Acts: The Power Continues

After the resurrection and ascension of Jesus, the Book of Acts tells the story of how miracles continued through the lives of his followers. The early church is marked not only by preaching and community, but by transformative power.

The apostles perform signs and wonders (Acts 2:43), healing the lame (Acts 3), raising the dead (Acts 9), and even surviving deadly snake bites (Acts 28). They are imprisoned and miraculously freed (Acts 5, 12, 16). Philip is transported from one place to another in a moment (Acts 8:40). Saul is blinded and healed (Acts 9), and his name was changed to Paul, a turning point in the story of the church.

These miracles affirm the continuing presence of the Holy Spirit—the same Spirit that empowered Jesus now lives in his followers. The miracles of Acts are not only a continuation of the ministry of Jesus; the miracles are also meant to be a sign that God's kingdom is expanding, reaching beyond Israel to include the Gentiles, beyond Jerusalem to the ends of the earth.

The Human Instrument: Faith as a Channel

Interestingly, when a biblical miracle takes place, a human is involved. God works through people—through Moses at the Red Sea, through Elijah calling down fire, through Jesus touching the leper, and through Peter healing the lame.

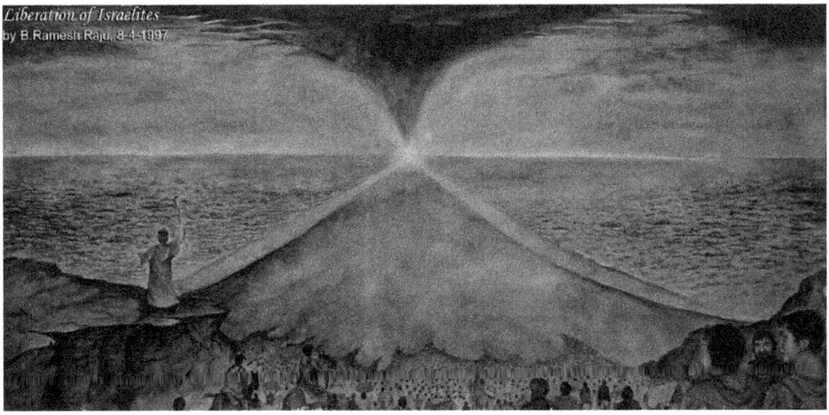

Moses parting the Red Sea, in Exodus 14. by B. Ramesh Raju (1997)
Public Domain made available under the Creative Commons CC0 1.0
Universal Public Domain Dedication. Wikimedia Commons

Why does God so often use human beings to perform divine acts? Perhaps because miracles are not only about power but about relationship. God invites us to participate in the sacred work of healing, delivering, and restoring. Faith, prayer, obedience—these are not levers to mechanically trigger miracles; instead, they are one way we align ourselves with God's will.

Jesus often said, *"Your faith has made you well"* (Mark 5:34). Our faith and trust in God open the door of our heart, mind, and spirit to receive the miraculous. Miracles reveal that God is not only above us but with us—and working through us.

Miracles East and West

While the Bible provides a rich tapestry of miraculous events, it is not alone. Across time and culture, the world's religious and spiritual traditions have recorded their own accounts of signs and wonders—testimonies to the presence of the divine in human affairs. These accounts, though differing in context and theology, share a striking resemblance in their power to inspire, heal, and transform (Kripal et al., 2024).

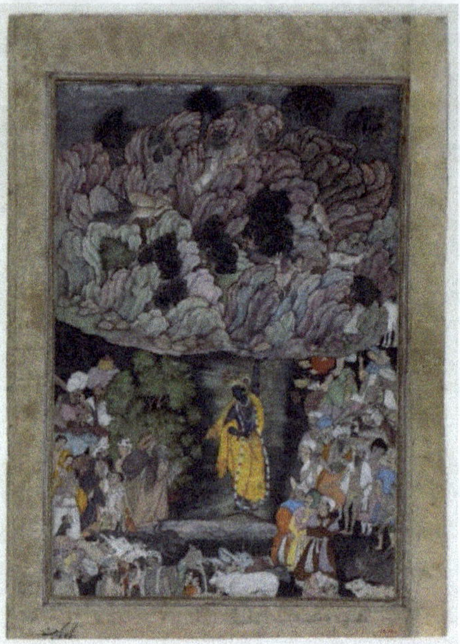

Krisha is depicted, in blue body, holding up a mountain with left arm to protect villagers. (1590-95) Attributed to artists at Lahore, Pakistan
Metropolitan Museum of Art, Credit line: Purchase, Edward C. Moore Jr. Gift, 1928; Object Number: 28.63.1
(The Metropolitan Museum of Art Open Access policy is: "you can freely copy, modify and distribute this image, even for commercial purposes").

Hinduism, one of the oldest living religions, abounds with miracles attributed to its many deities and holy figures. The *Bhagavata Purana* and *Mahabharata* tell of Lord Krishna lifting an entire mountain (Govardhan Hill) to protect villagers from torrential rains, and of sages performing feats through deep meditation and spiritual power. As Swami Vivekananda wrote, "The moment you fear, you are nobody. You become God the moment you have no fear," pointing to the belief that divine union unlocks God-like miraculous potential.

Buddhism recounts miracles in the life of the Buddha, such as his Twin Miracle, in which he emitted fire and water simultaneously from his body to address skeptics. The Buddha himself warned against the pursuit of miracles for their own sake yet acknowledged that profound spiritual attainments can manifest as extraordinary events. In the *Digha Nikaya*, the Buddha teaches: "Greater than any miracle is the miracle of instruction"—suggesting that inner transformation is the true marvel.

Islam honors the miracles *(muʿjizāt)* performed by prophets, especially the Prophet Muhammad. The Qur'an itself is considered the greatest miracle—the revelation of divine wisdom. Other accounts include Muhammad's night journey and ascension to heaven, and his ability to produce water, heal the sick, and even multiply food, as did Jesus. The Sufi mystic Rumi once wrote: "Don't you know yet? It is your Light that lights the worlds"—a reminder that miracles often emerge to awaken hearts.

In Indigenous traditions across the globe, miracles are experienced in close relationship with nature and ancestral spirits. Vision quests, healing rituals, and encounters with animal guides or celestial signs are considered sacred and transformative. Among Native American peoples, the appearance of the white buffalo is viewed as a miracle signifying hope and spiritual renewal. Australian Aboriginal dream stories are collected to preserve accounts of divine acts that shaped the land and gave it sacred meaning.

Contemporary interfaith dialogue has increasingly recognized that while human metaphysical frameworks differ, the longing for divine intervention, healing, and hope is universally human. Miracles, East and West, function as sacred symbols—threshold moments when the veil between heaven and earth lifts, offering a glimpse of the eternal.

Concluding Comments

Miracles, whether described in Scripture or through the sacred stories of many faiths—serve not to impress or dazzle, but to point—to point to something greater, deeper, and more enduring than spectacle. They invite us to ask: What is the source of this power? And how does it relate to us, today? The next chapter turns to these very questions, exploring how miracles are understood, encountered, and even debated in our contemporary world. The passage below from the New Testament lists "working of miracles" as one of the many gifts of the Holy Spirit. As we enter Chapter 17, How May Miracles Occur, we leave behind the ancient past—but not the mystery or the wonder that still calls to the human heart.

Below is a scripture that speaks of God giving people one or more spiritual gifts: to speak words of wisdom, share knowledge, impart faith, heal the sick, work miracles, discern spirits, to speak in tongues, or to interpret tongues as led by the spirit of God.

> **1 Corinthians 12:8-10:**
> For to one is given through the Spirit the utterance of wisdom, and to another the utterance of knowledge according to the same Spirit, to another faith by the same Spirit, to another gifts of healing by the one Spirit, to another the working of miracles, to another prophecy, to another the ability to distinguish between spirits, to another various kinds of tongues, to another the interpretation of tongues.

Questions to ponder:

- *What is you understanding of the miracles in sacred scriptures such as the Bible?*
- *Ever thought about why God would use human beings in working miracles?*
- *Have you experienced a miracle or visited a place or setting where a sacred miracle was said to have taken place?*

Chapter 17—How Miracles May Occur

Throughout human history, miracles have captured the imagination of believers, skeptics, and seekers alike. Often defined as events that transcend the laws of nature, miracles are typically understood as divine interventions that cannot be explained by science. But what if the framework of modern physics, particularly quantum mechanics, provide a bridge between the miraculous and the material? What if intention, prayer, and belief function not just as spiritual disciplines but as mechanisms through which reality itself can be influenced?

This chapter explores the intersection of spirituality and science, proposing that miracles may unfold through the interaction of three distinct but interconnected dimensions of reality: the material, the quantum, and the virtual levels.

The Three Levels of Reality

The Material Level: The Manifest Universe

Imagine reality as a vast structure composed of three levels or dimensions. The first is the **material level**, the everyday physical world perceived through our five senses. It is the realm of solidity, substance, and time—where mountains rise, rivers flow, and our body breathes.

Within the familiar material realm lies the **quantum level**, a realm of probability and possibilities, unpredictability and interconnectedness. Here, particles are believed to exist in multiple states simultaneously (superposition), can affect each other across vast distances (non-local entanglement), and behave differently depending on whether they are observed (by an interaction) or not.

And deeper still—beyond even time and space—is what we might call the **virtual level**. This is the dimension of pure information, universal consciousness, and divine intelligence. It is the source-code of the universe, the field of infinite potential, the dwelling place of what religious traditions call God.

Yet, these levels do not exist in isolation. They flow into each other like layers of a stream: the virtual informs the quantum, which shapes the material. Understanding how these levels interact may reveal the hidden mechanics of the miraculous.

The Quantum Level: The Realm of Possibility and Potentiality

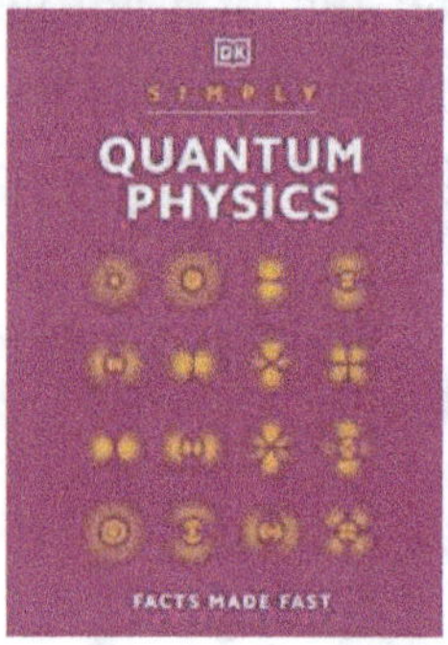

Dorling Kindersley, Ltd. is a British publisher that has joined with Penguin Random House to produce a 2025 best-selling book entitled, *Simply Quantum Physics*. The book is visually-focused with graphs, illustrations, and diagrams to explain the complex and abstract concepts of our physical universe. I can recommend it to anyone interested in learning more on the subject.

The universe, according to quantum physics, is not made of solid matter but of vibrating energy. Subatomic particles—the building blocks of atoms—are not fixed entities but probabilistic waves that blink in and out of existence, millions of times per second. In fact, 99.9999+% of what we perceive as solid is empty space filled with vibrating energy—held together at the atomic nucleus level by strong nuclear force which binds the protons and neutrons together, while electromagnetic forces hold the negatively charged electrons in their orbits. Also, the weak nuclear force influences the stability of atoms where quarks within protons and neutrons can change type—causing a proton to transform into a neutron or vice versa. At the atomic level, two or more atoms are held together by intermolecular chemical bonds and electrostatic forces. All this is taking place continuously in every moment throughout our universe and within our body, as well.

Predominately, cosmologists believe that at the moment of the Big Bang, all matter, space, and time were condensed into a **Singularity**—a point of infinite density and zero mass. From this singularity exploded the cosmos. As it cooled, quarks formed a cloud of particles which coalesced to form atoms, and atoms formed galaxies, stars, and ultimately organic life. The deeper one probes into this reality, the less solid it becomes. At the quantum level, nothing is fixed. Everything is potential. You and I were potential when a gleam came in the eye of our parents. Later, at our birth we became reality, yet always we are potential.

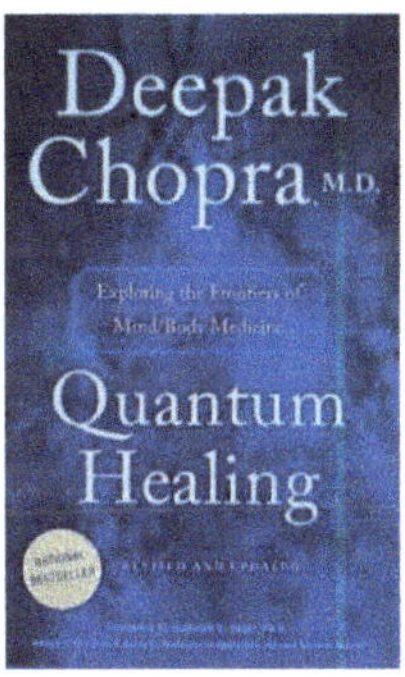

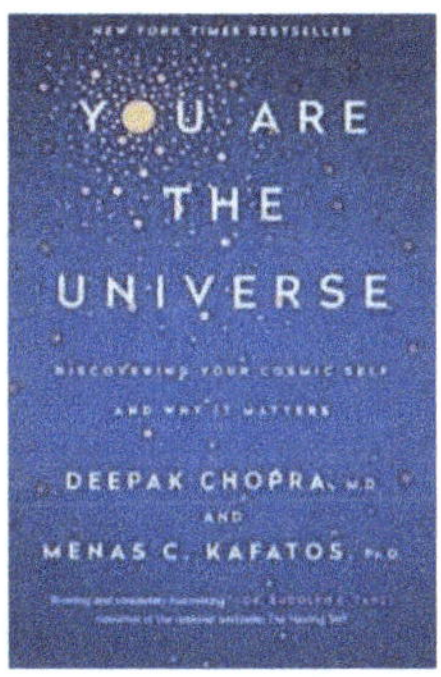

Potentiality is the key

The quantum realm is a place of pure possibility, and it appears to respond to human consciousness. Best-selling author and medical doctor, Deepak Chopra, has said: “If every atom and every molecule in the universe emerges from the quantum field, doesn’t this mean that our bodies do, too? Undoubtedly yes.” The statement, attributed to Chopra, encapsulates a central theme in his teachings: that our physical bodies originate from and are intrinsically connected to the quantum field.

Seeds of the miraculous

If our thoughts, beliefs, and intentions operate at the quantum level, then perhaps it is possible they can influence material reality. This opens the door to a radically new understanding of prayer and belief—not as hopeful wishes to a distant deity, but as **participatory acts of co-creation** that align human consciousness with the creative fabric of the universe and the ultimate will of The Source, God.

The Virtual Level: Consciousness, Intelligent Universe

Deep within or even beyond the quantum lies the virtual level. It is not virtual in the technological sense, but is a realm of information, consciousness, awareness, and intelligence. It is where the laws of nature are "written" before they are enacted. Here, words like Absolute, Universal, "consciousness," "spirit," and "God" begin to apply.

This domain may be what the mystics experience in moments of divine union, what saints tap into through deep prayer, and what visionaries describe as the ultimate source of creation. Quantum computers are being developed by harnessing minute spinning qubits at the inconceivably minute Planck level (1.6 X 10-35Meters). Yet, the virtual level may be felt when it flows into and with the vibrations of the quantum field and, from there, manifests in the material world.

The Power of Prayer and Belief

If we accept the possibility that the quantum field responds to consciousness, then prayer with firm heart-felt conviction becomes an act of co-creation. Numerous studies, including those conducted by researchers like Dr. Larry Dossey and Dean Radin, suggest that focused intention can have measurable effects—not only on the human body but also on random systems and biological processes.

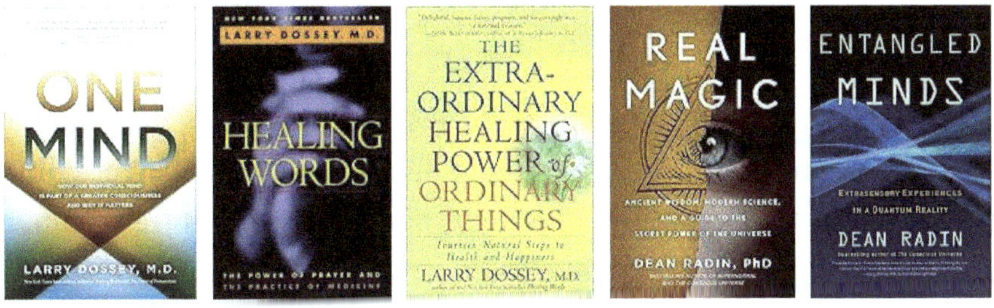

Even the placebo effect—long regarded as a medical curiosity—demonstrates the power of belief to influence the physical. When someone believes they will heal, they often do. This is not mere psychological trickery; it may be quantum causality at work. The conviction of the mind sends an intention through the quantum field, which then informs the material body.

Faith, then, is not a blind leap into the unknown, but an alignment with the deeper architecture of the created universe—where science and spirituality are both affirmed. It is aligning the human will to the divine frequency established at creation.

Biblical Miracles Revisited

Consider the miracles recorded in the Bible. From Moses parting the Red Sea to Jesus walking on water, these events seem to defy natural law. And yet, many of them involve a human intermediary—a prophet, a teacher, an apostle—whose faith and action trigger the miraculous.

Why would God involve humans in divine acts? Perhaps because consciousness is the conduit through which the virtual reality becomes manifest and real. Just as light passes through a prism and all the colors of the rainbow become visible, divine intention may pass through human intention to become reality.

Some notable examples:

- Moses striking the water to part the sea (Exodus 14)
- Jesus healing with a word or touch (Matthew 8, Mark 1)
- Paul and Peter performing healings and wonders (Acts 3, Acts 9)

Each instance suggests that miracles require more than divine will—they may also require human alignment. It is sobering to consider that many potentialities may not take place until a human being responds with belief and acts **co-creatively** within God's plan.

How Miracles May Occur: A Synthesis

When viewed through this tri-layered lens of reality, miracles are no longer supernatural anomalies—they are natural events occurring across all three dimensions of existence:

1. *In the virtual domain*, divine intelligence holds the blueprint of what could be.
2. *In the quantum field*, human consciousness (intention, prayer, belief) interacts with this blueprint.
3. *In the material world*, the result is an event that appears to defy expectation or probability.

Please understand, this is not a denial of God's role, but a deepening of it. God is not simply "out there," arbitrarily dispensing miracles. In my understanding, God is the source field of all reality, and human beings are invited to participate in that creative flow. More on co-creation in later chapters.

A Reflective Invitation

Has one of the Biblical or a present-day miracle especially captured your heart? Is there a story that resonates with something you've experienced?

And the point I wish to make is: what if the miraculous is not a distant relic of sacred history, but a present possibility for all? What if the next miracle waits not in the heavens, but within your own consciousness—ready to flow outward into the field of reality?

Perhaps the greatest miracle is not a suspension of the natural order, but the realization that we are already part of a greater order—one that listens, responds, and creates through us. Let those who have faith, believe; those who believe, co-create.

Concluding Comments

As we close this exploration into the nature of miracles, we stand at the threshold of a deeper truth: that a miracle is not just something that happens to us, but something that happens **through** us. When we align with divine intention, when we speak with faith, and when we move with conviction, we step into a role of **sacred participation**.

This brings us to the final chapter of Part III—Chapter 18, "Power of the Spoken Word." If the quantum field responds to belief, then the words we speak, imbued with certainty and integrity, may well carry a creative force of their own. Words shape perception, perception shapes energy, and energy shapes the world. As we continue, we will explore how speech, like prayer and intention, can channel divine authority to reshape both our lives and the lives of those around us.

Questions for thoughtful consideration:

- *What do you think about the 3 levels of reality—Material, Quantum, and Virtual?*
- *Science says the quantum level is one of possibility and potentiality. What does this say to us about our future?*
- *Are you able to appreciate how prayer with faith may affect the quantum level? Should this apply to how we pray?*
- *If this is true, what does this say about human responsibility and the ethical choices we make?*

Chapter 18—Power of the Spoken Word

"In the beginning was the Word, and the Word was with God, and the Word was God." (John 1:1)

There are few forces as underestimated by humanity as the spoken word. Nevertheless, from the ancient Biblical text of Genesis to the teachings of modern psychology, words have been recognized as vessels of immense creative and destructive power. In this final chapter of Part III, we explore the capacity of language—not just as a tool of communication, but as a sacred instrument of transformation.

The Word of God: A Creative Force

Hebrew scriptures open with a profound declaration: the universe itself began with a word. "Let there be light," God spoke—and light came into being. This idea is not metaphorical in the biblical tradition; it is literal. God speaks the universe into existence with the "Big Bang or the Big Breath."

The belief that the spoken Word is **generative**—that what is said makes things happen—is affirmed across spiritual traditions. It suggests that language, especially when spoken with faith and intention, can shape reality. To speak with conviction is to participate in the divine co-creative act. Our words are not merely an echo of a thought; they are sparks of possibility.

A Compelling Story

Not long after arriving to serve as a priest at St. Martin's Episcopal church in Houston, I received a phone call from a woman who attended my previous church. She asked if I would see her husband who had pancreatic cancer and was told medicine had nothing further to offer. Her husband's doctor said he had two or three months to live and being a relatively young man with two children he was distraught. A few days later they arrived in Houston, and when the man sat in my office chair, he immediately put his head in his lap, covering his face with both hands. He said nothing while his wife informed me of the latest information from his doctor including that he had been advised to get his affairs in order because he did not have long to live.

As his wife spoke, I continued to observe a man holding his head face-down in his lap. This touched me deeply for I could not recall seeing a man so emotionally captured by his sadness. I had no idea what I should say to him. So, I prayed silently, asking God for guidance. When his wife finished her update, what came to me was to tell him: "Sir, you appear to be a man who has lost all hope." Hearing this, he bolted to his feet and shouted, "Of course I have lost all hope! Didn't you hear what my wife said? I will be dead in three months!" I said nothing and he quietly sat back in his seat and put his head back in his lap. Moments later, I knew inwardly what I should say and was confident it was God's leading because what I had never said to any patient with cancer was what I was about to say to him. Yet, I believed I knew what God wanted him to hear.

I said, "Sir, before I became a priest, I was a physician, and in medical school I was taught that no cancer is one-hundred percent fatal, not even one that has spread throughout the patient's body." He looked up and I continued. "There is always a small percentage of patients who survive cancer even after medicine has given up on them." I told him that I recall my professor saying this is called a **"spontaneous remission."** By now the man was sitting upright and listening to my every word. I then said, "I know you, your wife, and the people in your church will be praying for you, and now that I have heard your story, I will be praying for you as well." I continued, "I believe you are going to have a spontaneous remission."

Immediately, the man's countenance changed, and a broad smile came across his face. He hugged his wife and embraced me. He was no longer the man who had entered my office and sat with his head in his lap. A transformed man stood before me aglow and rejoicing. He remained joyful as I walked with them to the parking lot and with a bright smile, he profusely thanked me for seeing him. He left, a man whose hope had been restored.

Years went by and, in the meantime, I had written a book entitled, *Graham Crackers and Milk: Food for the Heart and Soul*, which I thought would be soon on the best seller list—did not happen. But, I did have several boxes of books to distribute. I prayed about it and decided the people at my previous church would want a copy, so I arranged to go there. A book-signing date was announced in the church's bulletin. Twenty or so people showed up that day and I was busy signing books when the doors of the church swung wide open and the man I had not seen in years, entered shouting with arms raised, "Doctor Graham! I have raced across town at my lunch-break to let you know I am healed of cancer. Like you said I had a spontaneous remission! My doctors can find no sign of cancer in my body." Everyone clapped upon hearing of the man's healing. The next person in line said, "I need three of your books, please." Everyone laughed.

I have not received a further update on the man's condition. He may have been given three extra years to live (instead of three months), or he may be still alive today.

I tell this story with caution because I know people struggling with their own or a loved one's cancer could believe what they need to do is to pray for a spontaneous remission. Please understand this is not what I am saying or what you should hear. My assessment is that because I believed God had revealed what I was to share with this man and because he absolutely convinced that what I said was true, every cell in his body awoke with all the innate healing power within his body to put his cancer in remission. Had the man not accepted what I shared, I believe his cancer would surely have not gone into remission. In other words, I believe his remission occurred because he believed what God had me tell him was in fact going to happen. From that moment on he saw himself healed and his body responded accordingly. In religious terms, faith was translated throughout his entire being for healing. Furthermore, please understand, I have never mentioned the possibility of a spontaneous remission to another cancer patient because I have not felt God leading me to do so. Otherwise, I would give false hope to someone when that is not what they need to hear from me. I believe the important thing is to ask God what we are to say to someone who has cancer or another serious illness. Being present at a patient's bedside, holding their hand, and being with them may be God's perfect will for you and for them. Your presence and comforting love may be what is needed the most.

The "Miracle" of Words of Intent

Upon reading of the power of words and learning that our body is 70% water, a deeply religious Japanese businessman, Masaru Emoto (2007), sought to evaluate the effect of positive and negative words on glasses of water. His home-spun experiments were widely publicized in the press as proving that water exposed to positive words, emotions or music, formed beautiful, structured crystals when frozen, while water exposed to negative influence produced distorted and fragmental crystals. Emoto concluded that it is important to maintain an internal self-talk of positive thoughts and words concerning oneself and to maintain a healthy and harmonious environment. Also, being religious, Dr. Emoto proposed that the status of our internal water serves as a messenger between us and the divine, emphasizing our responsibility before the divine to maintain positive thoughts and actions for our well-being and that of others.

The problem is, Dr. Emoto was not trained in the scientific method and researchers quickly revealed there was little evidence that speaking to water could determine the structure of water when frozen. Nevertheless, social media articles continue to affirm that love represents the energy we wish to share, and gratitude is the energy we hope to receive, and declaring these two forces, love and gratitude, can create a powerful, harmonious balance that resonates with the fundamental structure of the universe. Others, emphasized cultivating love and gratitude in our lives creates a positive feedback loop of energy that enhances our sense of well-being and positively influences our environment. Finally, some mentioned that by understanding the interconnectedness of people and all aspects of our planet, cultivating love, gratitude, and harmony can potentially mitigate environmental and social issues.

Well said, but proving this scientifically is the problem. Kokubo et al. (2017) wrote an article discussing the methodology involved in water crystal research. The authors stated why Emoto's claims were insufficient from the viewpoint of modern science. There are many variables at work, including: the pH and temperature of the water, type and size of food particles, the number of bottles used, the "judges" chosen to assess crystal formation, as well as trying to control the methodology from lab-to-lab for repeatability. Proof in science is demanding, and it should be.

The Power of Spiritual Words

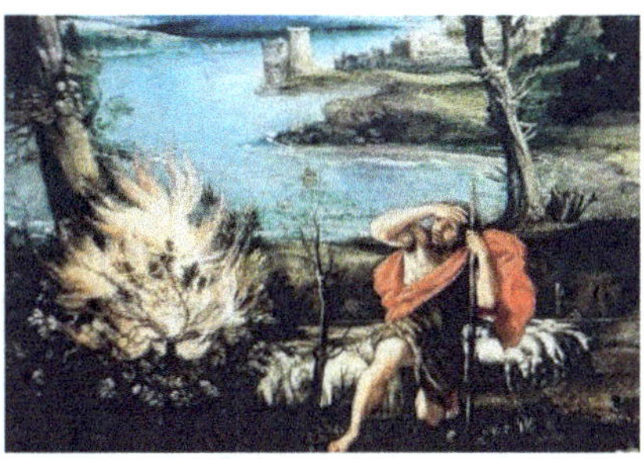

Moses and the Burning Bush, by Domenichino (1581-1641).
Public Domain made available under the Creative Commons CC0 1.0 Universal Public Domain Dedication. Wikimedia Commons.

As depicted in the painting above, in the book of Exodus (3:1-15), while tending a flock of sheep Moses saw a bush that was on fire but was not consumed by the flames. When Moses approached, God spoke from the bush telling him to remove his sandals because he was on holy ground. God then said, “I am the God of your father, the God of Abraham, the God of Isaac, and the God of Jacob.” Then, God told Moses that he was to go before Pharoh in Egypt and to lead the Children of Israel out of their bondage to their Promised Land. Hearing God wanted him to speak to Pharoh, Moses stammered and asked to know God’s name. God said: “I Am That I Am.” One can almost feel the authority that came forth when God spoke “I AM” and that name is all Moses needed to know. Out of reverence, the Jewish tradition does not speak aloud the sacred name of God and when written it typically has a hyphen, G-d.

Another Sacred Word is AUM

As a mantra, the word AUM has been used for thousands of years in Eastern religions and its use in the West is becoming more common. Typically, the mantra is used in the repeated chanting of the sacred word AUM. The word’s authority is said to come from it being the same word that was spoken by God at creation and therefore the word is believed to contain the vastness and energy of creation itself. To explain how repeated chanting of the word may lead to self-realization, Prophet & Prophet (2004), writing from a Christian perspective, state that to speak the Sanskrit word AUM means: “I bow, I agree, I accept . . . AUM! I accept the Lord God Almighty and I agree that I am his beloved son/daughter. I accept my immortal destiny. I accept my reason for being. I accept my responsibility to be. . .AUM.”

Affirmations of Faith in Religious Communities

In Christianity

Beyond sacred words for the name of God, words and affirmations of faith are spoken corporately during Christian worship services. Often the congregation will repeat together the Nicene Creed, a statement of faith focusing on the doctrine of the Trinity (God as Father, Son, and Holy Spirit) and the divinity of Jesus Christ. During the ordination of pastors and priests to the ministry, vows are made both by the individuals ordained and by the congregation to support the new minister.

There is a long tradition for couples who are married to repeat sacred vows while facing each other before a gathering of family and friends. Equally powerful is the service for the burial of the dead in Christianity, which begins with a powerful declaration: "I am the resurrection and the life, saith the Lord; he that believeth in me, though he were dead, yet shall he live; and whosoever believeth in me shall never die." Again, the authority of the statement is impactful especially if it is your loved one who has died.

In Judaism

In Jewish tradition, the blessing has significant power at weddings and funerals. At weddings, there are seven blessings recited during the ceremony and there is a prayer for fertility and prosperity. The common expression for good fortune, *Mazel tov*, and a toast to life, *L'Chaim*, are used to express well wishes at the reception where everyone raises a glass to celebrate. At funerals, "May (his or her) memory be for a blessing" is a common expression of condolence to honor the deceased.

In Islam

Specific words, phrases and verses from the Qur'an are considered powerful and are often cited in weddings and at funerals to invoke blessings. One such phrase spoken at weddings is "May Allah bless and unite both of you in goodness." The words and phrase are expressions of faith in Allah and are often used to make these and other important life events. One such powerful phrase is "Allah the merciful and beneficial."

In Eastern Religions

Eastern religions each have its own unique traditions for marriage and burial of the dead. Hindu weddings feature a rite where the bride and the groom tie a knot and take seven steps together around a sacred fire, one vow for each step. After the seventh, the marriage is considered complete. At death, Eastern religions include prayers, readings, chanting, and rituals to express their faith in the deceased's peaceful journey to their next stage of existence. Buddhist funeral ceremonies emphasize the importance of Karma and the cycle of rebirth with prayers, chanting, and offerings.

The Power of Spoken Prayers

In the event of an illness, in addition to seeking medical attention, it is common to express words in prayer to seek divine intervention to promote the healing process. Prayers can be said when a priest makes rounds in the hospital but more often prayers are said by the one who is ill, and among family and friends. Many churches welcome parishioners to come forward for healing prayer during Sunday services. Trained prayer teams are available to pray with those who request it or when a member requests prayer for a loved one or friend who is not present. Prayers are said for whatever the individual may need; for example, when dealing with interpersonal conflict, seeking employment, or preparing to move to a new city. At times the request can be, "Pray for me, I don't even know what to ask." Not only are prayers comforting, but they also give assurance that God has heard the request and many believe there is more power when more prayers are said. There are countless stories of the power of prayer.

Deepak Chopra, M.D., in his book, *Quantum Healing*, (2015) tells the story of Laura, a young woman who was diagnosed with breast cancer in her mid-thirties and elected not to undergo conventional treatment, despite her doctor warning without treatment she would be dead in less than two years. Chopra said, "Three years later she is still alive and appears perfectly normal. Her x-rays reveal that the tumor has not shrunk, but its growth has been slight." Although she is in remission, from a medical point-of-view her cancer is still considered present. Yet, Laura is pleased and believes she was right not to undergo traditional treatment for her cancer.

Journalist, Gina Ryder, in the June 09, 2022, issue of *Reader's Digest* published an article entitled "7 stories about the power of healing prayers." For example, Yamile McBride, a 40-year-old Educator in North Carolina, was suffering with exhaustion, low blood pressure, and irregular heart rate. This was distressing because her sister had undergone open heart surgery a year previously. After examination and tests, her doctor said she needed a cardiac pacemaker. The following Sunday, she shared her story at church and received prayer. Two months later, Yamile no longer had exhaustion, and her blood pressure and heart rate were normal. Her doctor said she did not need the pacemaker.

Another example of prayer and healing that was reported by Ryder is of 40-year-old Tara Geraghty whose three-year-old daughter began having breathing problems and was taken to the ER one night after it appeared she had stopped breathing. At this visit it was learned that her daughter had high-risk stage four cancer. She received chemotherapy, had a chest tube for weeks, and was on antibiotics for recurring infections. Tara says she prayed for her daughter like she had never prayed before. She put her name on every prayer list. After 78 days mom and daughter left the hospital, and her child continued to improve at home. Eight years later, at age 11, Tara's daughter is thriving and well. Tara is the creator of *"Cancer is Fun, New Jersey."*

A variation of the above stories is heard in most religious settings every week and for that reason many believe in the power of prayer to heal. Today, as with Tara's daughter, it is almost always a combination of medical science and prayer working together that can be said to be responsible for the healing. Indeed, **science and spirituality together are healthy companions**. People of faith often express thanks and gratitude to God for their physicians, nurses, and other caregivers, and typically view advancements in medical science as a divine gift to humanity. Finally, "the placebo effect" of prayer should not be discounted. Even when one does not believe in a divine intervention, belief in the power of prayer can initiate the healing response (The Placebo Effect in action).

Science and The Spoken Word

While written words may endure, it is spoken language that holds immediate transformative power in our lives. The tone, cadence, and intention behind our speech influence not only others but ourselves. We use words to express our emotions—love, anger, and hate. At the same time, we use words to express profound intellectual ideas and the principles underlying philosophy, law, theology and politics.

Neuroscience has shown that spoken affirmations can rewire neural pathways by a process known as neuroplasticity; conversely, negative speech can also rewire nerve pathways and generate stress hormones, adversely affecting health and one's emotional well-being.

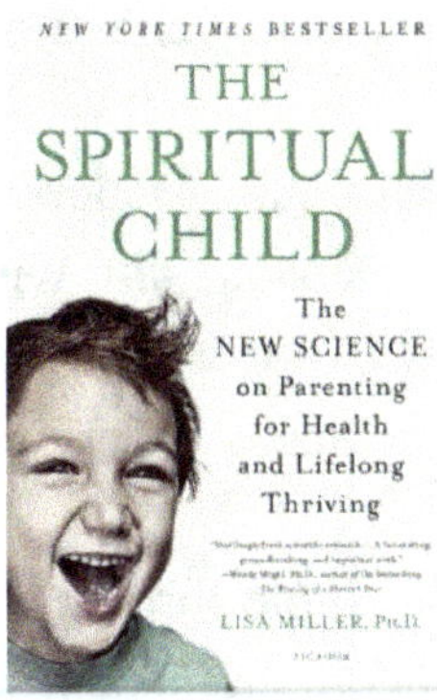

Columbia University, professor of psychology, Dr. Lisa Miller (2015), in her best-selling book, *The Spiritual Child: The New Science on Parenting for Health and Lifelong Thriving*, addresses the power of positive and negative words spoken and heard during childhood and as an adult, especially from those who have power in our lives—our parents, teachers, and friends. Miller says, words matter because they construct our internal narrative. They become the scripts we live by. Telling a child, "You are loved and capable," becomes a seed that may flourish into a life of purpose. Telling them, "You'll never amount to anything," can become a self-fulfilling prophecy of limitation.

Psychoanalysis Zvi Lothane (2007) has addressed the power of the spoken word in everyday life, in psychiatry, and psychoanalysis stating that words are the essential tool of mental treatment. Yet he says it is often difficult for laymen to believe pathological disorders of the body and mind can be eliminated by "mere words." Words however are important because they are the means psychotherapists use to create mental and emotional transformation.

For this reason, Lothane says psychotherapy could be called **"word therapy"** because its efficacy comes from the power of suggestion, the influence the therapist has upon the patient by means of the spoken word. He says in life "the most important interpersonal action and emotion is love, feeling love, and expressing it, among others, in words." Almost magically, love words can have a healing effect. You may think you are being asked to believe in magic and to Lothane, that is not far from the truth.

Throughout history, religious leaders have stirred nations, comforted souls, or incited chaos—all with words. Jesus calmed storms and healed the sick with a word. The prophets called for justice with fiery proclamations. The apostles spread the gospel with inspired speech.

Our everyday words, too, ripple through the quantum field. When we speak truth, love, and encouragement with conviction, we may be activating hidden dimensions of reality—just as prayer and intention influence the quantum level. Speaking becomes a spiritual act, a declaration that aligns our energy with the source of creation.

Concluding Comments

As we close Part III, we stand with new awareness of the unseen forces that shape our world. We have explored the dimensions of reality—the material, the quantum, the virtual—and seen how prayer, belief, and intention may activate the miraculous. Now, we recognize that our voice, too, is a channel of divine influence.

To speak with authority and conviction is to speak from alignment with truth. It is to become a vessel through which the power of the Word continues to create, bless, and heal. Whether in prayer, affirmation, encouragement, or proclamation, our speech has the potential to reframe our lives and the lives of others.

As you move forward, stay mindful of the language you use—not only in public, but in the quiet moments when you speak to yourself. Let your words be rooted in love, confidence, and sacred intention.

And now, having explored the miraculous, the quantum soul, and the power of belief, we turn our attention to a new horizon: Eternity. In Part IV, we will delve into the mystery of what lies beyond this life—drawing upon near-death experiences, spiritual accounts, and the profound question of life after death. If miracles are glimpses of eternity breaking into time, then perhaps death is not an end, but a threshold. Let us cross it with open hearts.

> **Matthew 17:20:**
> He said to them, "Because of your little faith. For truly, I say to you, if you have faith like a grain of mustard seed, you will say to this mountain, 'Move from here to there,' and it will move, and nothing will be impossible for you."

Questions to ponder in reflection:

- *When Moses asked God for his name, God said: "I Am That I Am." Any thoughts about the meaning of the phrase I AM? Can you feel the authority it holds?*
- *In the story a man with cancer given 3 months to live, believed he would have a "spontaneous remission" and received at least 3 extra years of life. What are your thoughts?*
- *Any thoughts about the Hindu/Buddhist traditions and the sacred word AUM? Can you see it as representing the breath of God at creation?*
- *Lisa Miller's book, The Spiritual Child, speaks to the importance of words of affirmation to a growing child. What are your thoughts about the power of the spoken words a child may hear at home, and school, and on the playground?*

PART IV: ETERNITY

Introduction to Part IV: Eternity

As we now turn the final page of this journey, we enter the mystery that has captivated the human spirit since the beginning of time: **Eternity**. Part IV of this book is dedicated to exploring what lies beyond the veil of physical death. This section seeks to delve into spiritual, religious, philosophical, and experiential perspectives on life after death—especially insights emerging from near-death experiences (NDEs), mystical encounters, and other paranormal phenomena that offer glimpses into the eternal.

In the previous three parts, we explored **Belief, Mystery, and Miracles**. We examined how beliefs evolve over time, how mystery is essential to a spiritual life, and how miracles—far from violating the laws of creation—may emerge from deeper laws not yet fully understood. We reflected on the miraculous nature of existence itself, particularly the phenomenon of life on this planet. These explorations laid the groundwork for the transition into our final theme: the enduring question of what awaits us after our earthly journey.

Eternity is not merely a theological idea. It is a deeply personal subject, requiring courage, openness, and spiritual imagination. We approach it now with humility and hope.

Eternity

He who binds to himself a joy
Does the winged life destroy
He who kisses the joy as it flies
Lives in eternity's sunrise.
Poem by William Blake (1757-1827)
Public Domain, Wikimedia Commons

Chapter 19—Eternity Defined

What is **eternity**? To begin to answer this question, we must step back—far back—to the origin of everything. Nearly 13.8 billion years ago, the universe is believed to have emerged from a single point in an event known as the Big Bang, or as I and others now call it, the **Big Breath** (from the Mind of God). From this explosion of radiant energy, space and time were born. From cosmic dust, stars were born, galaxies coalesced, and planets formed. Among them Earth—our fragile blue home.

And yet, even this grand narrative is but a prelude to the idea of eternity. For if all matter, all energy, all time itself emerged from a singularity, then eternity must lie beyond it (prior to the Big Breath). Eternity is not simply a very long time. It is a condition outside of time—more a state of being, rather than a measure of duration. As a state of being, eternity is present always—now and after our death.

Cosmologists speak of a universe destined for eventual entropy: a slow fading into stillness. But the soul, many of us believe, is not bound by entropy. It is bound for something beyond the limits of physics—a divine dimension of continuation, reunion, and purpose.

Van Gogh: At Eternity's Gate

Willem DaFoe's Academy Award-nominated performance as Vincent Van Gogh in the movie, *At Eternity's Gate*, presents the story of an artist we all know and love today. He also was a man who had a tormented soul. Psychiatrists and neurologists have identified at least a dozen mental illnesses that could have been the source of his agony. In particular, the possibility of him having temporal lobe epilepsy which may explain his spells of self-rage, anger, despair, and self-mutilation. Even Vincent's last words expressed the grief and rage he experienced in life: "Grief is eternal" (Taghipour et al., 2019).

Nevertheless, Simon Schama, in his book *The Power of Art* (2006), depicts van Gogh as a beautiful example of one who was able to embrace both his art as well as his faith in God. This explains van Gogh's hope that his art would awaken viewers with the divine power and light of the epiphany. Many of Vincent's letters to his brother Theo, express his union of art and faith including a letter in which he said: "God, it's beautiful. The world I mean. Sunlight. Sunflowers. The faces of ole women. Gnarled hands. Night skies. Cypresses in the wind" (Smee, 2018).

A Personal Reflection

Several years ago, my wife and I led a group from our church to view religious art in Italy and France. While in southern France, we visited Saint-Rémy-de-Provence where Vincent spent a year in a mental hospital. We were told when the director of the hospital learned that van Gogh was an artist, he told Vincent to take his easel outside and paint scenes around the hospital. Van Gogh's brother Theo kept him supplied with paint, brushes, and canvas. Vincent painted over 150 of his most beloved paintings, including *The Starry Night* (1889). and paintings of wheat fields, olive groves, sunflowers, and irises. A few days later, on our hotel rooftop, with wine glasses held high, we shouted to the heavens: "Vincent van Gogh, despair no longer, you and your paintings are beloved by everyone today!" We hoped he heard us as we sang and with all our hearts we shouted again and again, "We love you Vincent." After leaving the mental hospital, still in the grip of despair and having sold only one work of art (to an aunt), Van Gogh committed suicide at age thirty-seven. Everyone on our tour was deeply touched by Van Gogh's story, and on our hotel rooftop we sang Don McLean's song entitled "Vincent" and again shouted, "We love you, Vincent!"

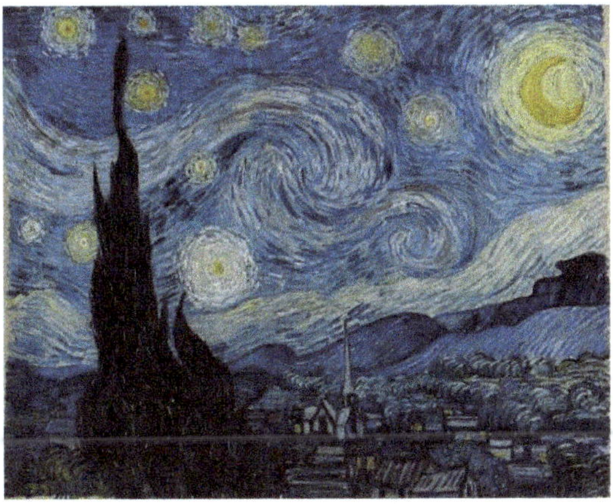

The Starry Night, Vincent van Gogh (1889), Museum of Modern Art Wikimedia Commons, This work is in the public domain in the United States because it was published (or registered with the U.S. Copyright Office) before January 1, 1930.

Facing Death: Fear of the Unknown

Despite the lofty metaphors used by St. John to describe heaven as having twelve pearly gates and streets of gold (Rev. 21:21), fear and uncertainty surround the topic of death among Christians and people of every culture and faith. The unknown is unsettling, and death—the great unknown—can provoke dread, anxiety, and avoidance. Yet, across spiritual traditions, we find words of comfort that can soothe this fear and provide assurance.

Wisdom from World Religions

The soul is understood to be ever-unfolding. As the Bhagavad Gita says: "The soul is neither born, and nor does it die. It was not brought into being, and it will not cease to be. It is eternal and everlasting" (Prabhupada, 1983).

Christianity

Jesus offers profound reassurance in the Gospel of John (14:1-3):

> Do not let your hearts be troubled. You believe in God; believe also in me. My Father's house has many rooms; if that were not so, would I have told you that I am going there to prepare a place for you? And if I go and prepare a place for you, I will come back and take you to be with me that you also may be where I am.

This passage is often read at funerals, and with good reason. It speaks directly to the human fear of being forgotten, lost, or alone after death. Jesus paints a picture of eternity not as an abstract place, but as a home—a realm of welcome and belonging.

Dr. Wolfgang Achtner, Professor of Theology at the University of Giessen and a leader in the dialogue between science and religion, offers a Trinitarian view of eternity and time that resonates with both spiritual tradition and contemporary insight. In his perspective, eternity is not static but a dynamic, ongoing expression of divine action—creating, sustaining, redeeming, and renewing the unfolding of time. Each Person of the Trinity plays a distinct role in this sacred continuum: God the Father initiates and upholds the fabric of time through creation; God the Son, through the crucifixion and resurrection, redeems time and works across history to renew humanity; and God the Holy Spirit, as the divine creative force, inspires and guides transformation within the stream of history. The future, in this vision, is not fixed but emerges as a field of *open possibilities*—an idea that echoes the quantum indeterminacy discussed earlier in this book. Achtner emphasizes that human consciousness, when joined with the Holy Spirit through faith, can actively participate in shaping the present within God's redemptive plan.

Although Achtner's work may sound too theological, I personally appreciate his recognition of God not as a controlling autocrat but as a loving and creative force, actively involved in all that is taking place in the eternal now. This is a view of God who is imminently present in all aspects of our moment-by-moment life on planet earth and in the afterlife which we all will experience. A loving God is there too.

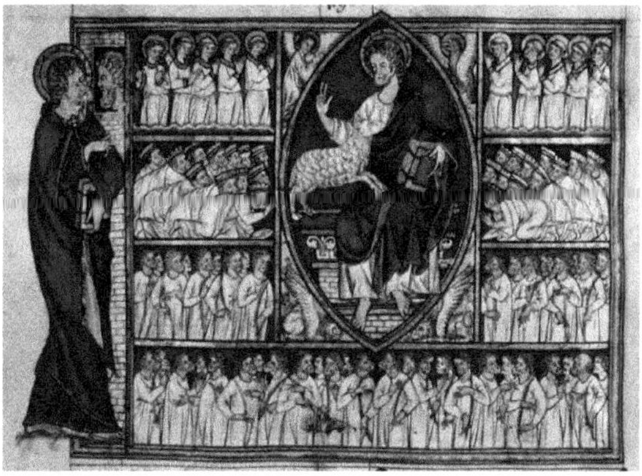

Revelation 7:9-16

"After this I looked and there before me was a great multitude that no one could count, from every nation, tribe, people and language, standing before the throne and in front of the Lamb. They were wearing white robes and were holding palm branches in their hands. And they cried in a loud voice: 'Salvation belongs to our God, who sits on the throne.'"

An Illuminated Manuscript of the Revelation of St. John, *The Apocalypse*, created for Edward I and wife Eleanor of Castile (Anonymous, prob. 1270). Public domain, Wikimedia Commons.

Islam

The mystical tradition within Islam has struggled with the traditional understanding of Allah (God) as being totally transcendent and not imminent as in Judeo-Christianity. However, within Islamic mysticism mentions waqt, time, to express the notion of timelessness and eternity as an attribute of Allah. Sufism also mentions a peak experience known as Ibn al-waqt that is free from the past and the future—the Eternal Now of God.

Hinduism

The yoga approach to understanding and experiencing time and eternity is identified with immortality and Brahman (God). In yoga, respiration corresponds to an eternal time influencing internal rhythm of the body and its organs. The breathing practices in yoga lead to awareness of the unreality and illusion of time which is interpreted to be an activity of ego. In deep meditation, one's higher consciousness has no illusion of past, present, or future. Only the present moment, now, exists.

Buddhism

Buddhism is about ending suffering, achieving enlightenment, and attaining nirvana with teachings that focus on the practice of Meditation, the Four Noble Truths (suffering, its cause, cessation, and the path to it), the Eightfold Path (right understanding, thought, speech, action, livelihood, effort, mindfulness, and concentration), and the Five Precepts (moral guidelines for ethical living). A core teaching from early Buddhism is that of "universal instantaneity" which affirms the **interconnectedness and impermanence** of all phenomena. This means that everything, including humanity, is constantly in a state of flux, in an unending cycle, and that each event or being is linked to all others. The concept that everything in the universe is interconnected is recognized in quantum physics as mentioned elsewhere in this book. Ultimately, the goal in Buddhism is to achieve Nirvana.

Nirvana is not a place to go after death; rather, it is a state of enlightenment and liberation from the cycle of rebirth and suffering. Nirvana is a state of being, characterized by the understanding of the true nature of reality, the cessation of all suffering, and the absence of attachment. As a state of being, Nirvana can take place in the present moment for those who are alive and enlightened.

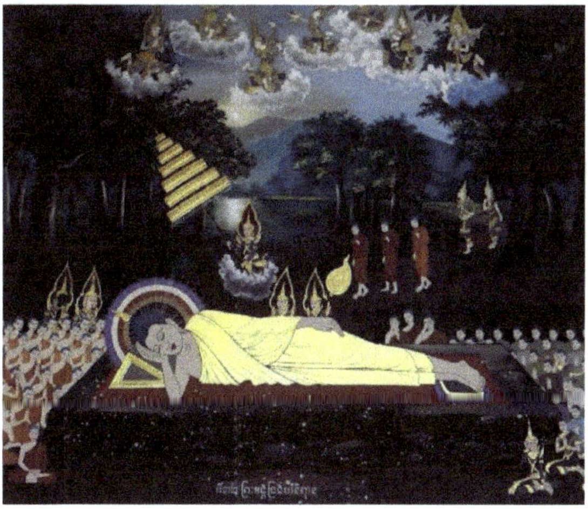

Mural of Gautama Buddha Priv Nirvana by Chanrasmey Miech, in Cambodia. Wikimedia Commons, Public Domain licensed under the Creative Commons Attribution-Share Alike 4.0 International license.

Zen-Buddhism and Taoism

The three aspects of traditional Buddhism—the mutual entanglement of all being, the connection of being and time, and the emphasis on the present moment as the ultimate reality—also play an important role in the Zen-Buddhism and Taoism. While all three, Buddhism, Zen-Buddhism, and Taoism, share similarities in their focus on inner peace and understanding, they differ in their origins, core philosophies, and practical approaches.

Zen-Buddhism emphasizes direct experience and insight through meditation and mindfulness. It speaks of an aspect of time as pure presence which can open the door to trans-temporality, among Japanese Zen-Buddhists this is called Nikon. **Trans-temporality** is the idea that all moments in time exist simultaneously—past, present, and future. This is explored in quantum science, particularly in relation to the quantum theory of time, which suggests that time is not a linear flow but rather a structure where all events are equally real. The time we measure with our wristwatch and calendars is a helpful necessity for ordering daily life, but it is not reality. Einstein said the past and the future are illusions; only the present moment exists.

Taoism is a Chinese philosophy and religion which focuses on living in harmony with the Tao, which is understood as "the Way" or "the Path." To achieve balance in life, Taoism focuses on naturalness, simplicity, and effortless action (wu wei). This isn't laziness but being authentically natural and spontaneous, while simplifying life. Taoism embraces the **interconnectedness** of all things while viewing humanity as part of the universe's whole. It also affirms spiritual immorality where the human spirit (qi, energy) rejoins the universe after death, becoming part of the universal energy of the universe. The spirit becomes one with the Tao, a state of harmony and unity with the universe. Putting it another way, the ultimate Way or Path (Tao) for the individual spirit is to be absorbed back into the natural order.

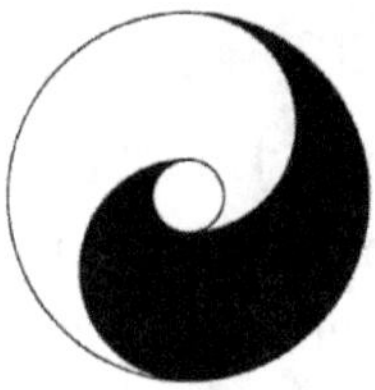

Original Yin/Yang Symbol, by unknown author from the Zhou Dynasty period. Symbol in Taoism for balancing energy.
Wikimedia Commons, This work is in the public domain because it consists entirely of information that is common property and contains no original authorship.

Indigenous Traditions

Indigenous beliefs about eternity and life after death vary widely by tribe, but a common thread is the belief in a spirit world or afterlife where the deceased continue to exist. Many Indigenous culture's view death not as an end, but as a transition to a new stage of existence, often within the spirit realm or the journey to another world. Many depict the spirit world as a place in the sky where their deceased ancestors have gathered and continue to live, free from pain and suffering. Basically, death is viewed as a part of life and a transition to a new life. Almost all indigenous groups have rituals and ceremonies that are meant to guide the deceased in their journey to the afterlife where they will be reunited with tribal ancestors.

Respect for All Creatures

Upon the death of an animal, the indigenous tradition is to view an animal as sacred and their death is observed with respect and gratitude, often with rituals and ceremonies. Many believe that animals, like humans, have a soul and can be reborn. Taking an animal's life for food is viewed as necessary but done with reverence and recognition of the animal's death as a sacrificial gift, the shedding of blood. Indigenous cultures often believe in the interconnectedness of all living things and that each creature, all things, and all aspects of creation are essential to maintain a balance in nature. That being true, the message is to only take what is needed from nature and without the exploitation of resources.

Great Spirit Prayer

Oh, Great Spirit,
Whose voice I hear in the winds
and whose breath gives life to all the world.
Hear me! I need your strength and wisdom.
Let me walk in beauty, and make my eyes
ever hold the red and purple sunset.
Make my hands respect the things you have made
and my ears sharp to hear your voice.
Make me wise so that I may understand
the things you have taught my people.

Let me learn the lessons you have hidden
in every leaf and rock.

Help me remain calm and strong in the
face of all that comes towards me.
Help me find compassion without
empathy overwhelming me.
I seek strength, not to be greater than my brother,
but to fight my greatest enemy: myself.
Make me always ready to come to you
with clean hands and straight eyes.
So when life fades, as the fading sunset,
my spirit may come to you without shame.

Translated, Lakota Sioux Chief Yellow Lark (1887)
https://archives.library.umaine.edu/repositories/2/resources/3583

Unity in Principle

In world religions there is a general commitment to a belief in the value of unity and the interconnectedness of all things. As to ethics, almost all religions affirm The Golden Rule, respect all life, and have their version of the Ten Commandments—respect for the divine, and not to murder, steal, or defame others. Together, the corporate world views offer a mosaic of hope, transcending doctrines and echoing a universal truth: death is not the end, but a threshold.

Unity in Practice

All traditions affirm the importance of engaging in practices to cultivate a deeper spiritual life. Below are listed three types of spiritual practices that are recommended almost universally:

- Withdrawal from worldly distractions to focus inward (meditation, contemplation, prayer, mindfulness, retreat).

- To engage in regular bodily wholeness exercise to strength will power (Pilates, walking in nature, yoga, or tai chi).
- The use of a breathing practices (deep breathing, abdominal breathing, box breathing, alternate nostril breathing).

The goal of these practices is to engage one's whole person—body, mind, and spirit—and to open one's mind and heart to discover one's true Self and, by grace, to encounter the divine presence, The Source, Ultimate Reality, God.

God and Eternity

Craig (2001) begins his book entitled, *God, Time, and Eternity* by observing that the Jewish God, YHWH, "never came into existence, nor will God ever cease to exist." In other words, as creator of the universe, God has always existed, was always present at and before creation, and will continue for all eternity—beyond when the universe will cease to exist.

In Christianity, eternity refers to God's timeless existence and the future state of humanity. In traditional Christianity, eternity continues for humanity after death either in Heaven with God (eternal life) or in Hell (eternal damnation). Although eternal life is not guaranteed for all human beings, provision has been made for everyone to enter eternal life by choosing to accept God's gift of salvation through the life, death, and resurrection of Jesus Christ (Ephesians 2:8-9).

However, the New Testament epistle, 1st John 2:2, says, "He (Christ) is the atoning sacrifice for our sins, and not only for ours but also for the sins of the whole world." While not traditional Christian theology, today many Christians take the passage literally and reject the concept of eternal damnation proclaiming, 'God is a God of love,' and therefore all will be saved. Although the concept that all will be saved is attractive, this view has not been accepted by most Christians, principally because, in this understanding, the gift of eternal life must include those considered evil (the Adolph Hitlers of every generation). Most will question this by saying that the God of love is also the God of Justice.

In Judaism, God is said to always be present everywhere, as the Psalmist has beautifully expressed:

> Where can I go from your Spirit?
> If I go up to heaven, you are there.
> If I make my bed in the depths,
> If I rise on the wings of dawn,
> If I settle on the far side of the sea,
> Even there your hand will guide me,
> And your right hand will hold me fast. (Ps. 139: 7-10)

Psalm 139 is comforting when one approaches the end of life or upon the death of a loved one. The Psalmist is saying that we are not alone. God is always there, even at the point of death and the divine presence will be with us following our death as well.

Eastern and Western Views

In the Eastern spiritual traditions, eternity is often framed not as a linear progression of time, but as a cycle. Life, death, and rebirth form the wheel of samsara, through which souls reincarnate again and again until they reach Nirvana, liberation from the cycle and union with the eternal.

In Western traditions, particularly within Christianity, Judaism, and Islam, eternity is understood more linearly. Life leads to death, which leads to an eternal state—whether union with God in heaven or reincarnation. Both perspectives, though different in structure, affirm a sacred continuity beyond death.

Human beings across cultures share a longing for this continuity. In a letter to Countess Margot Sizzo-Noris-Crouty, January 23, 1924, poet Rainer Maria Rilke wrote, "The great secret of death, and perhaps its deepest connection with us, is this: In taking from us a being we have loved, death does not wound us without also lifting us toward a more perfect understanding of this being and of ourselves."

We humans want to believe that life does not end. That our consciousness, our unique presence in the world, is not extinguished but transformed. Yet, life is so filled with grief it is hard for some to hold a positive view of life after death. As we saw earlier, Vincent van Gogh may have been an example of this.

Final Reflections

In my own ministry, I have had the privilege of leading a Bereavement Support Group for over twelve years. I have seen the face of grief transform over time into the light of healing. I have heard many stories of dreams, signs, and mysterious encounters that indicate an ongoing connection with loved ones who have passed.

In Chapter 12, we explored over **fifteen ways to navigate uncertainty**—through breathing practices, meditation, retreats, yoga, and more. These same tools can help us face death with greater peace. When we are spiritually grounded, death does not always feel like a cliff but can be seen more like a crossing.

Concluding Comments

To summarize, eternity is a mystery but one we can glimpse through revelation, scripture, intuition, and love. The longing for it—the sense that something beyond this life endures—is woven into the human soul. Whether through ancient scriptures, mystical experiences, or the assurance of one's faith, eternity continues to beckon.

In the next chapter, we will go deeper into the nature of **Human Consciousness**. What is the soul? How does consciousness relate to the body and the brain? Is consciousness confined to this lifetime, or does it persist beyond death? Before moving on, it may be worthwhile to sit with these questions:

- *Van Gogh's art is beloved today, yet it was rejected by people in his own day. Do you believe the rejection of his art had a negative effect on his mental illness and suicide?*
- *In the book of Revelation in the Bible, heaven has streets of Gold and pearly gates. Do you view this literally true? If not, how do you view heaven.*
- *World Religions paint a positive picture of life after death, yet many people have a fear of death. Why do you believe many people of faith have a fear of death?*

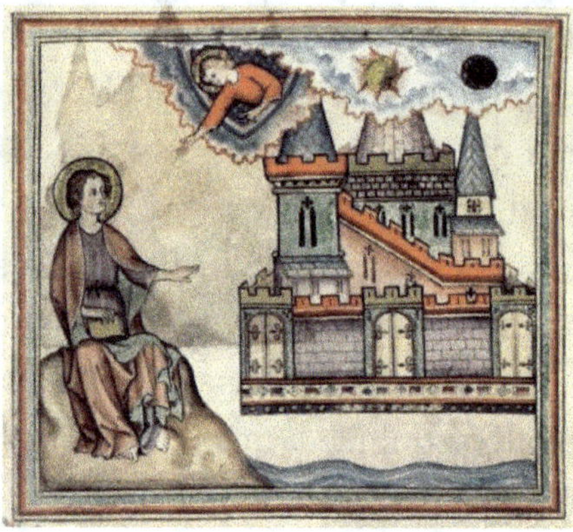

Depiction of The New Jerusalem coming down from Heaven in the book of Revelation 21 (1330 CE). When St. John wrote the book of Revelation he visualizes heaven as a place of purity, clarity, and divine beauty. Wikimedia Commons. Public Domain in the United States because it was registered before January 1, 1930.

Chapter 20—Human Consciousness

Human consciousness is the lens through which we perceive Eternity and everything else. In many ways, the nature of human consciousness is **the core mystery of existence**. It is the seat of our thoughts, our self-awareness, our memories, our ethics, and our experiences of beauty and pain. Yet despite its centrality, consciousness remains one of the greatest mysteries of science. Award-winning author, columnist and editor, Stephen Schwartz (2021) writes:

> What is consciousness? What is information? Those, to me, are the two great mysteries. After 50 years of experimentation research studying consciousness, I have come to this conclusion. Max Planck and many of his colleagues in the German school who created modern physics were correct. Consciousness is causal and fundamental. Spacetime arises from consciousness not consciousness from spacetime. It is not a new idea, but today, we are able to use experimental science to test our ideas about it.

Plato and Aristotle

Before considering the current science of consciousness, let's look at two ancient beliefs about the nature of consciousness. In the 4th century BCE, Plato and Aristotle debated about the material and spiritual dimensions of reality. **Plato** envisioned a world of unchanging Forms that exists separate from the physical world. **Aristotle**, on the other hand, considered the soul to be the inseparable from the body. In other words, Plato believed in a dualistic reality, with Forms as the ultimate reality, while Aristotle focused on the material world as the single, primary source of reality. Plato's belief in a separate soul and body, led some early Christians including Justin Martyr and Augustine of Hippo to proclaim Plato to be a "proto-Christian."

St. Augustine and the Seeds of Potentiality

In view of current scientific thinking, insight concerning consciousness that came from St. Augustine, bishop of Hippo (354-430 CE) is amazingly before its time. He described creation as existing in "seeds of potentiality"—hidden sparks of life and purpose embedded in the cosmos, awaiting their unfolding. He also proposed that creation was, in essence, a thought in the mind of God. In this vision, reality itself is not an accident or a byproduct of random chance, but an intentional act of the Divine. Seeing creation as a thought in the mind of God, some have said the Big Bang is best understood as the Big Breath (e.g., of God). Genesis 1:3-28 we read, "And God said, 'Let there be light, and there was light."

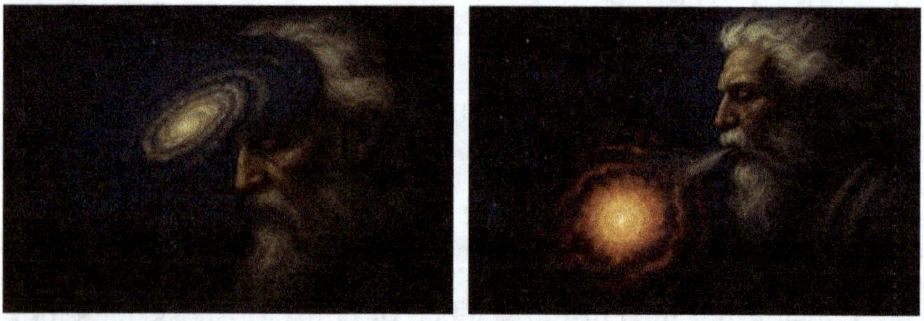

AI depictions of the Universe as Divine Thought and The Big Breath at Creation

If the universe is, at its foundation, a divine thought—then consciousness is not merely a byproduct of biology or our brain. Instead, consciousness is part of the very fabric of reality. This means, each of us, in our conscious awareness, reflects a glimmer of the divine mind. Our lives, our experiences, our ability to know and to love, are not accidents in a cold universe. They are the flowering of those ancient seeds—growing in time and pointing beyond it.

The Big Bang and Fine-Tuning Revisited

As we return briefly to the moment of **creation**—the Big Bang—we are reminded of the **fine-tuning** of the universe. From the precise strength of the laws of physics to the delicate balance of fundamental forces, the conditions necessary for life are extraordinarily specific. Even a minuscule variation in the physical constants would make life as we know it impossible.

For some, this fine-tuning is coincidence. For others, it is evidence of a **cosmic intelligence**—an awareness, a mind, a consciousness—that is not only behind the origin of the universe but also an ongoing Presence within it. The great spiritual and philosophical traditions have long proposed that **consciousness precedes matter**. Science may still debate this, but the question remains open: is consciousness an emergent property of the brain—or is the brain a receiver of something greater, consciousness?

The Mystery of Consciousness

What is consciousness? At its most basic level, it is **awareness**—of self, of others, of time and space. It includes the capacity to think and reason, to feel and imagine, to be self-aware. Our understanding of consciousness ranges from being fully awake to a lesser alert state of consciousness—such as focused awareness, and other states including meditation, mystical union, dreaming, and the unconscious. With an intentionally quietened mind, relaxed body, and measured breathing, individuals report the experience of timelessness, peace, oneness, and encounters with the divine.

Despite centuries of inquiry, science still cannot fully explain the source of consciousness. Where does it come from? How does the subjective experience of consciousness arise from the firing of neurons? These are the so-called "**hard problems**" of consciousness. Some suggest consciousness is an illusion; others propose it is a fundamental force, like gravity or time. Some profess belief in panpsychism where all matter—organic (animals & plants) and inorganic (rocks, water)—is conscious (because all matter has an atomic structure and all atoms have nuclei and electrons that obey the fundamental laws of physics). Some mystics say they can feel the vibration of an inanimate rock or stone, implying the stone has life. Indeed, there is energy within the atoms that make up a stone or rock.

Are Plants Conscious?

Whether plants are conscious is typically dismissed by pointing out that plants do not have a brain or nervous system; therefore, a plant cannot possibly have conscious awareness. Yet, the question really is, can we determine if plants are conscious when we cannot explain consciousness within the animal kingdom on Earth? For centuries native cultures have honored and given thanks for plants that provide food (fruit and vegetables) to eat, and for the wood of trees to build canoes for transportation and a dwelling. Today, we value plants for the gift of photosynthesis that converts sunlight into energy and releases the oxygen we breath, and for herbs, bark, and mineral oils that provide chemicals for drugs and medicine to fight illness. And who would want to live on a planet like Mars that has no foliage? The question of whether plants have conscious awareness was addressed in 1848 by German physician, Gustav Fechner, in his book *The Soul Life of Plants*, and more recently by Tomkins & Bird's (1974) in their best-selling book, *The Secret Life of Plants*.

Although no one can give a definitive answer to the question of whether plants have consciousness, it is worthy of consideration. If for no other reason, surveys reveal 50% of people believe they communicate with plants. I have a relative who said he planted a bush that should flower but didn't for three years. Disappointed, he firmly let the plant know he was giving it one more year, and if it didn't blossom, he was going to cut it down. The plant responded with an abundance of blossoms and the man believes the plant "heard" his warning and blossomed to stay alive. He is not alone in believing communication with plants is possible.

So, what would it require scientifically to indicate plants have conscious awareness? First, plants are living organisms composed of organic matter. They are vital to the world's ecosystems and food chains. Like humans, plants are communal and reproduce sexually, where male and female gametes combine to form seeds and pollinate by being distributed by wind, water, insects, or other animals to new locations where the seeds germinate and grow into new plants. Plants also reproduce asexually, termed vegetative propagation, where parts of a vegetable—roots, stems, or leaves—can create new plants. Humans help the process by grafting and hydroponic techniques. Plants interact with other plants and adjust to environmental changes, soil conditions, and disease. When touched, exposed to sound, or lovingly cared for by a human, plants have been shown to alter their growth pattern and the color of its leaves and blossoms. There is evidence that plants communicate between each other through their roots and are able to warn neighboring plants of the danger of invading insects or when adverse weather is approaching. It has been reported plants are able to starve the roots of unwelcomed plants that threaten to steal their water and material resources. More recently, Kirlian photography has been used to capture images which show a blue haze or corona around leaves, petals, and stems of plants. This is said to represent the plant's energy, aura, or life force. Finally, many believe plants have conscious awareness and intelligence because, like human beings, plants have a double-helix DNA in the cell's nucleus that orchestrates cellular function as it does in all living things. The next time you smell a rose, be sure to express appreciation to one of God's most beautiful creations, and the gift of life plants are for us.

Neuroscience and Consciousness

Understanding how consciousness arises from neural activity remains one of the biggest challenges for neuroscience. Over 30 years ago, Crick & Koch (1990) challenged neuroscience to discover a theory to explain consciousness. As of today, although four main theories have been proposed none is widely supported. A major problem is that everyone has some idea of what is meant by consciousness, yet at any moment we are unaware of most of what is going on in our brain (e.g., the unconscious). Consciousness has been broadened to include animals who clearly experience some aspects of consciousness—ants, birds, whales, dauphins, monkeys, chimpanzees, gorillas, and elephants all have communication skills with others in their species. Even one-cell organisms have DNA with a rudimentary consciousness and are smart enough to flee from toxic environments. As mentioned above, plants also have cell structure and are believed to communicate with other plants through a connected root system. This means consciousness can no longer be limited to higher animals, as previously thought. Furthermore, when scientists attempt to measure consciousness, the question of subjective qualia arises—are two individuals seeing the same color "red" or not?

In a review of the cognitive science literature on consciousness, Jimenez et al., (2025) have focused on **the problem** of measuring subjective experience. They state:

> The central issues that make the study of consciousness so challenging is that, while the rest of science is concerned with problems that can be verified from a **"third person"** view (i.e., objectively), the study of consciousness deals with the phenomenon of subjective experience, only accessible from a **"first person"** view.

Two approaches have been used in the study of consciousness—objective (performance based) and subjective (report based) measures of awareness. In their article, Jimenez et al., (2025) evaluated both approaches in consciousness research and state often the attempt is made to transform a first-person experience-based report (subjective, subject to observer's judgment) into objective performance third-person observations that can be measured. For this reason, researchers have dismissed subjective methods and embraced what are felt to be objective methods to assess awareness. However, although objective methods offer the advantage of being third-person they do so by an indirect measure of the subject's true awareness. Furthermore, validity has been questioned for both the subjective and objective approaches. Nevertheless, robust research continues, and multiple theories have been proposed to explain the origin of human consciousness.

Four Scientific Theories of Consciousness, and More

In an extensive review of the literature, Yaron et al. (2021) identified four theories that have substantial empirical and theoretical interest among neuroscientists. They are: Global Neuronal Workspace (GNW), Higher-order thought (HOT), Integrated Information Theory (IIT), and Recurrent Processing Theory (RPT). GNW proposes that conscious processing emerges when information is globally broadcasted by a frontoparietal network, while HOT ascribes consciousness to higher-order representations in dorsolateral prefrontal cortex. Conversely, IIT claims that a maximum of power likely resides in a posterior cortical "hot zone". Finally, RPT asserts that horizontal connections and recurrent loops between lower and higher-level brain areas underlie conscious processing. The theories differ in their core principles, suggested mechanisms, and predictions they make about neural activity associated with consciousness.

In addition to the four theories mentioned above, from the Neurological Institute for Research and Treatment (IRCCS) in Milan, Italy, Sattin et al., (2021) screened 20,443 articles that address human consciousness. This was narrowed to 81 full-text articles which received a thorough three-step "scoping" analysis offering over 70 theoretical models for consciousness. Each gave its own definition which collectively provides a broad definition for consciousness. This study identifies the multitude of approaches that scientists have used to identify the source of human consciousness. The vast majority are focused on the brain and nervous system as the source of human consciousness, generally locating sensory input from the five human senses to various areas of the brain (prefrontal cortex, cingulate cortex, parietal cortex, temporal lobe, or occipital cortex, Thalamus, Limbic system, hippocampus, brain stem, and cerebellum). Recently, studies have included quantum theories emphasizing sub-atomic particles in the pre-frontal cortex and microtubules of the brain. Science remains focused on materialism and most scientists, but not all, have largely avoided any consideration of the brain serving as the receiver or translator rather than creator of human consciousness. So, let's consider the concept of a beyond-the-brain consciousness, an intelligent universe as the source of human consciousness.

Human Consciousness and the Intelligence of the Cosmos

From a spiritual standpoint, consciousness is understood not to be a byproduct of the brain but as **a reflection of the soul and spirit** connected to **Universal Consciousness** (God). Furthermore, many mystics and sages affirm that we are not just conscious beings—we are consciousness itself. Most believe when the body dies, consciousness continues.

Best-selling author, Gregg Braden (2025) has written:

> The scientific discoveries of the last 150 years, such as the mysterious result of the double-slit experiment, showing how invisible waves of potential energy collapse into the visible particles of reality when we observe them, have already shown that **consciousness, reality, and belief are intimately related**. They also have shown that our brains and bodies are wired with nerve cells that enable us to make use of, and participate in, that relationship. The ability to use consciousness to navigate the field that connects all things is a perfect example of a modern-day application of this ancient relationship that spans consciousness and our everyday world.

An Intelligent Universe. Ervin Laszlo, one of the foremost thinkers bridging science and spirituality, presents a vision of the universe that is intelligent, interconnected, and purposeful. In The Intelligence of the Cosmos, Laszlo outlines eight propositions as to who we are and why we exist. At the core of his theory lies the belief that human consciousness is not a byproduct of the brain—instead, consciousness is received, translated, and integrated into our being by our brain. "The cosmos is not a blind, indifferent mechanism. It is a living, evolving intelligence—and we are its conscious expressions" (Laszlo, 2017).

Laszlo's Credo—eight propositions summarized for clarity and for thoughtful consideration:

1. The cosmos is infinite and eternal intelligence.
2. This intelligence gave rise to a finite space-time reality: *the universe*.
3. All observed phenomena are clusters of vibration, "informed" by cosmic intelligence.
4. At varying frequencies, these vibrations become matter, mind, and intuition.

5. All forms—matter and consciousness—evolve through space and time.
6. Matter evolves toward super-coherence; consciousness evolves toward love and unity.
7. The universe serves to receive and transmit the intelligence of the cosmos.
8. The ultimate human purpose is to consciously foster this divine transmission.

The Universe is a Field of Vibration. Modern quantum physics has arrived at the view that space is not empty but a plenum field teeming with vibrational potential—multiple fields within fields of energy. Electromagnetism, gravity, and nuclear forces emerge in this quantum field. Laszlo suggests that consciousness itself arises from—and reflects—this deeper field of intelligence.

In his theory of the Implicate Order, quantum physicist Daivd Bohm has said, "Space is not empty. It is full, a **plenum** as opposed to a vacuum, and is the ground for the existence of everything, including ourselves" (Rodriquez-Rosello, 2019). Bohm's concept of space is it being a vast sea of energy that underlies all of reality. In other words, we are part of an ocean of energy that makes up the universe.

The Brain as a Receiver, not a Generator. Laszlo asks: *What if the brain is a receiver of consciousness, rather than its source?*

To use a familiar metaphor, compare the brain to a television set: it does not create the program, but it receives and displays it. Similarly, human consciousness may be a projection of something more fundamental: the infinite and eternal intelligence of the cosmos, received by our brain.

Prophetically, Nicola Tesla said, "The day science begins to study non-physical phenomena, it will make more progress in one decade than in all the previous centuries of its existence."

A Divine Mirror: When the Universe Sees Itself

In this light, human consciousness becomes more than an individual experience—it becomes a cosmic mirror. Through it, **the universe views itself**. The intelligence (God) that created the cosmos has intentionally become conscious by remaining present within creation itself.

13th century mystic, Meister Eckhard said, "The eye through which I see God is the same eye through which God sees me." And 20th century astronomer, cosmologist and astrophysicist Carl Sagan said, "We are the universe experiencing itself." In this view, creation is not merely something God created in the past—the universe is something divine intelligence continues to experience in and through our every act of awareness.

An Illustration: The Flow of Intelligence and Consciousness

The Source → Universal Consciousness → Human Consciousness → Choices

Interestingly, the flow can also be represented as a **loop**—because as we become aware, reflect, and pray, we feed intelligence back into the cosmos (like a mirror, quantum information and consciousness goes in both directions—meaning, the Source is aware of all choices):

Choices → Human Consciousness → Universal Consciousness → The Source

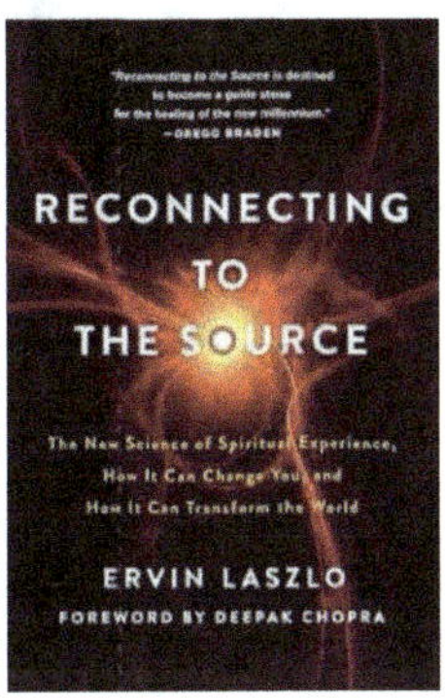

In his book, *Reconnecting to the Source*, Ervin Laszlo (2020) writes:

> The cosmos which is the ultimate ground of 'being,' is wholeness-oriented and wholeness-orienting. It inspires love and belonging among and between all things. This insight is the core of spiritual experience. We are, or can be, loving beings in a love-oriented world. If we fail to live according to who we are and what the world is, we have only ourselves to blame.

Sacred Participation: The Divine Act of Becoming

If this vision is true, then every moment of thinking, moving, acting, and loving becomes an act of sacred participation. In contemplating beauty, seeking truth, or offering love, we are not just passively observing the universe—we are **co-creating** it. If the term co-creation disturbs you, I will address this in an upcoming chapter.

Persian mystic poet Hafiz (1320-1389) said, "I am a hole in a flute that the Christ's breath moves through—listen to this music."

To awaken is not merely to know—it is to reveal and express the intelligence that gave rise to us.

Power vs. Force

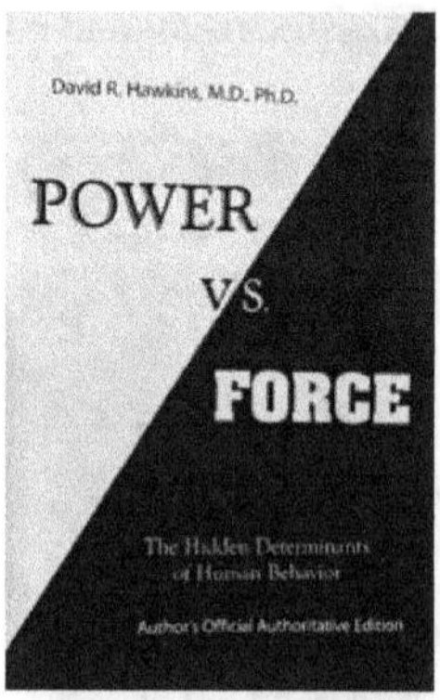

David Hawkins, M.D., Ph.D., has written a book entitled, *Power vs. Force: The hidden Determinants of Human Behavior* (2012) which contrasts the use of power and force in human relationships. Force divides because of the use of coercion and commands that cause counter-reaction, conflict, polarization, and disunity. Conversely, true power unites because its energy is spirit and the essence of spirit is to respect, honor, and aligns with the energy of life itself. Force equals weakness, lack of life, and death.

Hawkins's book includes a **Map of Consciousness**. It is a great resource to evaluate one's own life but also that of institutions, organizations, religions, and nations. In Hawkins's book are chapters revealing the impact of consciousness on athletics, politics, creativity, health and wellness, as well as tools to embrace Truth and meaning in life. It also includes guidance as how to measure the level of Truth and of consciousness.

Final Reflection

Ervin Laszlo's insights resonate with both ancient mysticism and the latest discoveries of physics. Neither asks us to abandon reason nor does it ask we jettison our faith community—but to deepen it. Consciousness is seen as a sign—a sacred sign pointing beyond to the depths of reality, inviting us to awaken, to participate, and to become whole.

Concluding Comments

Consciousness is the threshold between the physical and the eternal. As St. Theresa of Avala has imagined, it is the inner "cathedral" of our being, connecting to the presence of a divine mystery we cannot fully grasp, yet deeply sense. The more we listen to it, the more we discover that we are not alone. We are part of something far greater.

Let's now journey on to Chapter 21: Universal Consciousness, The Mind of God, after pondering these questions:

- *Why has it been so difficult to explain consciousness which we experience every day?*
- *Do you believe plants and animals have consciousness? What about a tiny ant? A rock?*
- *Any thoughts about the Divine* Mirror—*that the Universe* (God) *views itself through us?*

Chapter 21—Universal Consciousness, The Mind of God

The more we explore human consciousness, the more we are drawn into something greater—a shared awareness, a sacred presence that seems to permeate all existence. In this chapter, we will explore the profound idea of **Universal Consciousness**—what some might call the **Mind of God**—and its implications for how we live, relate, and understand ourselves and the cosmos.

A Second Look at Human Consciousness: The Mirror of the Soul

Before pondering universal consciousness, let's return to consider human consciousness, the miracle by which we experience life. It encompasses awareness, thought, perception, memory, and the remarkable ability to reflect on our own existence. Through **self-awareness**, we become not only observers of the world, but participants in it—co-creators capable of shaping reality with our intentions, thoughts, and actions.

Consciousness manifests across a spectrum of states—from alert wakefulness to sleep and dreams, from altered states induced by meditation or trauma to moments of transcendence. Practices such as **prayer, meditation, contemplation, yoga, tai chi, and mindfulness** help cultivate deeper awareness. They offer pathways to stillness and expanded perception—places where the boundary between self and world begins to blur.

It is in these quiet spaces that many experience a connection to something greater, an awareness beyond their own mind. This leads us naturally to the idea of **Universal Consciousness**.

Universal Consciousness: The Web That Connects All

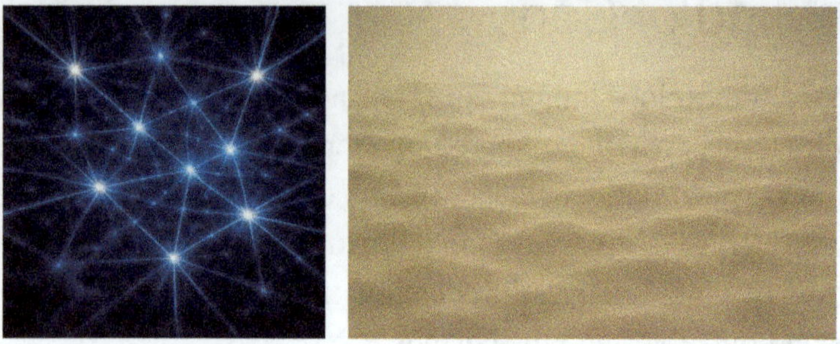

AI's effort to depict the Universal Quantum Field, Vibrating at the Speed of Light, interconnecting all things

Universal Consciousness is the philosophical and spiritual concept that all beings and all of creation are interconnected through a shared awareness. It suggests that consciousness is not isolated within individual minds, but flows through all existence—binding galaxies, plants, animals, and people in an invisible tapestry of unity.

This concept echoes across traditions:

- **In Christian theology**, we are members of one body, animated by God the Spirit.
- **In Eastern philosophy**, the self is not separate but a manifestation of the divine whole.
- **In science**, some quantum theorists suggest that consciousness may be understood as a field, like gravity or electromagnetism, woven into the very structure of reality.

If we are indeed part of a universal consciousness, then what we do to others, we do to ourselves. This has profound implications for **ethics and morality**. Harming another being—human or otherwise—is not simply an isolated act; it reverberates through the whole. Conversely, acts of kindness, compassion, and justice uplift the whole.

Sacred Texts and the Voice of Unity

The sacred writings of the world are filled with echoes of this truth—reminding us of our inherent unity with one another and with God (Kripal, et al, 2024).

Self-Awareness and Reflection

Psalm 139:23–24

"Search me, God, and know my heart… Lead me in the way everlasting."

> This prayer acknowledges the role of divine presence in human self-reflection. It affirms that awareness is not just psychological but spiritual.

Romans 12:2

"Do not conform to the pattern of this world but be transformed by the renewing of your mind."

> This points to consciousness as a vehicle for spiritual transformation. The renewal of the mind leads to a new way of being.

Interconnectedness of All

1 Corinthians 12:12–14

"Just as a body, though one, has many parts… so it is with Christ."

> Paul speaks of a shared spiritual identity that unites diverse individuals into one living organism.

John 17:21

"That all of them may be one, Father, just as you are in me, and I am in you."

> Jesus envisions unity not only among believers but between humanity and God—an indwelling communion that transcends separation.

The Upanishads
"Tat tvam asi"—You are That.

> This statement affirms the oneness of the self (Atman) with the universal spirit (Brahman).

The Heart Sutra (Buddhism)
"Form is emptiness, and emptiness is form."

> This teaching reflects the interdependent nature of all things. Nothing exists in isolation; everything is part of a deeper unity.

Collectively, these sacred insights point us to the same horizon: that our consciousness is not ours alone. It is a wave on the ocean of universal being.

Living with the Awareness of Oneness

When we embrace the reality of universal consciousness, we can no longer live as though we are separate from the rest of creation. We begin to see the face of God in the stranger, the cry of the earth in ecological injustice, the divine spark in every encounter.

This awareness calls us to live differently—to act with compassion, to seek justice, to care for the planet, and to honor the sacredness of every life. It is not enough to believe in God; we are called to live as participants in the **Mind of God**, where love, truth, and unity prevail.

A Holographic and Information Universe

Current scientific research is exploring what is known as the **cosmic hologram** or **holographic universe**. Stephen Hawking discovered that black holes radiate thermal energy. Other researchers believe that the total information content of a black hole is stored on the surface of the event horizon of the black hole. It was soon realized holography could not be applied only to black holes. Recently, the idea of a holographic universe added to a mixture of wormholes, quantum entanglement, and quantum computers. Information is required to describe the complexity of such a system.

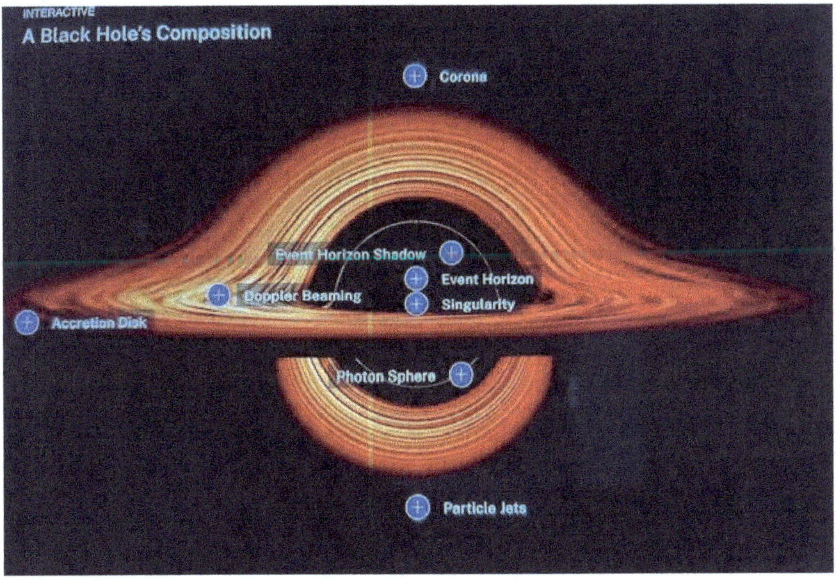

Black Hole Event Horizon. image credit: NASA's Goddard Space Flight Center Research Astrophysicist Jeremy Schnittman, Public Domain

The Holographic Principle

As to the holographic principle, (Rodriguez-Rosello, 2019) basically states that our three-dimensional universe—filled with galaxies, stars, planets, houses, and people—is a holographic image of reality that is projected on a distant two-dimensional surface. As stated previously, the holographic idea was inspired by the understanding that in the case of a black hole, the information content of all the objects that fall into the hole is still believed to be intact and contained in surface fluctuations at the black holes event horizon. In any case, a holographic universe is compatible with interconnectivity and wholeness.

The unique thing is a holographic picture, or hologram, captures and reproduces the entirety of a three-dimensional scene, not just a two-dimensional representation like a photograph. Holograms encode information about the light field of an object, allowing us to see the object in 3D, including depth and perspective, when viewed. In other words, we see in whole, not in part. What has this got to do with universal consciousness?

Theoretical Information Universe Theory

The Intelligent Universe (Chestney, 2024) is called the Theoretical Information Universe theory which states that **information**, not energy or matter, is the fundamental building block of reality. Much like our computers quantized information as binary digits or bits (0 and 1), so too at universe's most basic level—Planck level (1.6x10-35M)—our Intelligent Universe has qubits that convert information to energy and vice-versa. Unlike classical bits, **qubits** are not restricted to being in a definite 0 or 1 state. A qubit is a fundamental unit of quantum information that exists in superposition which is capable of both states 0 and 1 spinning at the same time. Every sub-atomic elementary particle can encode one qubit with spin-up or spin-down states (information). The outcome is probabilistic, determined by the qubit's state at the time. How does the transformation from qubit information to energy take place? Physicist Federico Faggin (2024) writes:

> There are irreversible atomic transformations that transform quantum information (entangled qubits representing experience or meaning) into live information that can in turn be represented with classical symbols (bits). This is the mechanism by which meaning is converted into live information and vice-versa.

Faggin suggests the universe can best be understood as a vast information processing system where everything (and everyone) is encoded as information. Energy and information are viewed as interchangeable. In fact, the mass of an electron (from Higgs field), the energy it possesses, and its position in space are all considered to be encoded information. Encoded information is applicable to the function of a single-cell paramecium to a complex multi-organ human being with 50 trillion cells.

Today, we have entered a technological "quantum revolution" enabled by quantum information and soon, quantum computing will literally revolutionize every aspect of the world we live in. In 2022, Nobel laurate Anton Zeilinger said: "What I believe but cannot prove is that quantum physics requires us to abandon the distinction between information and reality." In other words, Zeilinger wishes he could abandon any discussion of Information theory when talking about reality but knows he cannot. In fact, quantum information is now recognized as a fundamental quality in physics, like energy or matter.

Jude Currivan and The Cosmic Hologram

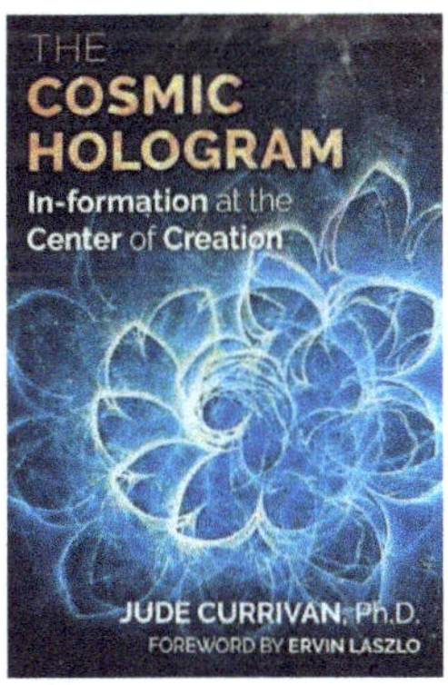

In her book, *The Cosmic Hologram: In-formation at the Center of Creation*, physicist and cosmologist, author, and lecturer, Jude Currivan (2017) writes:

> The growing scientific perception of the informational nature of all that we call physical reality is, at the same time, showing it to be in-formational. In other words, our Universe is composed not from arbitrarily accumulated data and accidental processes, but ordered, patterned, relational, meaningful, and intelligible in-formation, exquisitely balanced, incredibly co-creative, staggeringly powerful, and yet fundamentally simple.

Currivan also says there cannot be an in-formed universe without the existence of an in-former. She goes on to say, "The inevitable question that these scientific revelations come to is: Who or what is the **ultimate intelligence** that makes our perfect Universe?"

When we ponder an intelligent holographic universe, our interconnectedness and fundamental unity and oneness, the perceived separation between mind and matter becomes meaningless and the dilemma can finally be resolved with an understanding of the all-pervasive unity and wholeness of all-encompassing universal consciousness, the mind of God.

Concluding Comments

Human consciousness invites us to explore the mystery of our own awareness. But **universal consciousness** enlarges our understanding of the nature of God and reveals that we are never alone in that journey. We are part of a divine mind, a cosmic intelligence that surrounds, sustains, and calls us into deeper communion.

In the next chapter, we will explore some of the most compelling evidence of this shared awareness—stories from those who have glimpsed the other side through **Near-Death Experiences**. These accounts offer not only hope, but insight into what it means to be fully alive, fully conscious, and eternally connected.

First, these questions to consider thoughtfully:

- *Universal Consciousness is the concept that all beings and all of creation are interconnected through a shared awareness. What do you think about this?*
- *If all things, all creatures, and all human beings are interconnected, what does this say to us about our moral responsibility to our planet and to others?*
- *If information is created at the Planck level by multi-dimensional spinning qubits where all is probability, do you have any thoughts or implications that come to mind?*
- *What are your thoughts about being a co-creator with God?*

Chapter 22—The Near-Death Experience

Among the most intriguing and transformative experiences reported by people of all cultures and faiths are Near-Death Experiences (NDEs). These are profound psychological and spiritual events that often occur when a person is near physical death or in a state of extreme trauma. While interpretations vary based on cultural and religious context, the core elements of NDEs are strikingly consistent—and they raise profound questions about the nature of consciousness, life, and what lies beyond.

There are many accounts suggesting what lies beyond this life, including that of Dr. Eben Alexander, a neurosurgeon who, at age fifty-four, was unconscious in a coma for seven days due to a rare illness. In his book *Proof of Heaven: A Neurosurgeon's Journey into the Afterlife*, Dr. Alexander explains that although the cortex of his brain was non-functioning during this time, he experienced a reality in which consciousness is "completely free of the limitations of the physical brain." This suggests that death is not the end of consciousness. Alexander asserts that consciousness "continues under the gaze of a God who loves and cares about each one of us and about where the universe itself and all the beings within it are ultimately going" (Alexander, 2012).

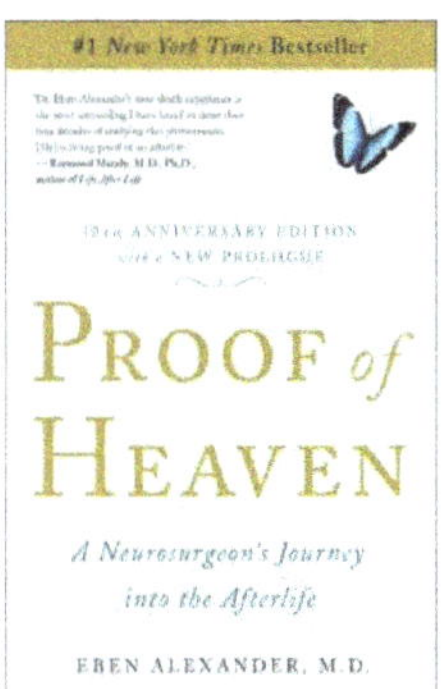

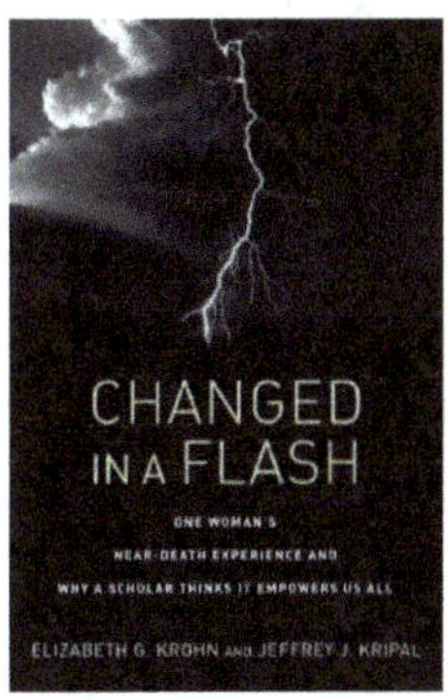

A Compelling Story

Some years ago, my wife and I attended a talk at the C. G. Jung Center in Houston, where a woman, Elizabeth Krohn (2018), shared the story of her near-death experience, which was later published in a book entitled, Changed in a Flash. Her presentation left a deep and lasting impression on both of us. At the time we heard her speak, Elizabeth was a woman in her mid-life, calm and grounded, but the experience she recounted had occurred many years earlier when she was a young mother raising two boys.

The occasion was a memorial service for her grandfather at their synagogue. As she pulled into the parking lot with her children, a sudden and torrential rain began to fall. She told her older son to run ahead and take cover under the veranda, then picked up her younger son in her arms and stepped out into the storm. In that instant, a bolt of lightning struck her.

She collapsed beside the car, lifeless. But what she described next was extraordinary.

She found herself walking—not in her body, but as if she were somehow outside of it— moving towards the veranda. When she got there, no one paid any attention to her. Then she noticed people were running in the rain toward her car. That's when she saw her own body lying on the ground, and several men hovering over it.

Then, she began to rise.

She described entering a tunnel, with a bright light in the distance, that opened into a breathtakingly beautiful space. The colors of the flowers were unlike anything she had ever seen, radiant and shimmering. There was a pervasive sense of serenity and a peace deeper than anything she had ever known. She saw people walking about, their faces beaming with contentment and joy.

And then, she said, God came and began speaking to her not in words, but mind to mind.

She described the encounter as warm and deeply personal. They spoke what felt as if it lasted half an hour. Then came a moment of choice. God told her she could remain in that realm or return to her earthly life. It was entirely up to her.

She thought of her boys, still so young, and chose to return.

Before she did, God told her three things would happen. First, she would feel intense pain when she re-entered her body because of the lightning strike. Second, she would go through a divorce—something she had not anticipated. Third, she would one day give birth to a daughter, a child she had always dreamed of having.

She re-entered her body, and the pain was immediate and overwhelming. Paramedics arrived, and she was taken to the hospital. When she told her husband what had happened, he dismissed her saying: “You always were crazy.” Not long afterward, he filed for divorce.

But life moved forward. She remarried and, just as she had been told, gave birth to a baby girl.

For many years she kept her experience to herself, sharing it only with her children. Her ex-husband’s reaction had made her cautious. But over time, she began to hear stories from others—people describing their own near-death experiences with strikingly similar details. She realized she was not alone, and that it was time to share.

When she gave her talk at the Jung Center, two of her three children came to support her. Now adults, they confirmed everything she said. They had heard the story when they were young, and it had never changed. They, too, were pleased to learn that other people had experienced something similar.

My wife and I found Elizabeth to be sincere and credible, and her story resonated with truth. It was a profound example of the near-death experience—not only as a moment of spiritual awakening, but as a turning point in the mystery of life, death, and what lies beyond. We have since shared her story with our own family and friends. And we also invited Elizabeth to share her story as part of a panel discussion on NDE at the Institute for Spirituality and Health.

The Near-Death Experience

Today, many articles have been appeared in the literature in which men and women share their stories of having had a near-death experience. Not all have the same experience, of course, but what they do share are among these eight things listed below that most have reported happening.

1. Out-of-Body Experience (OOBE)

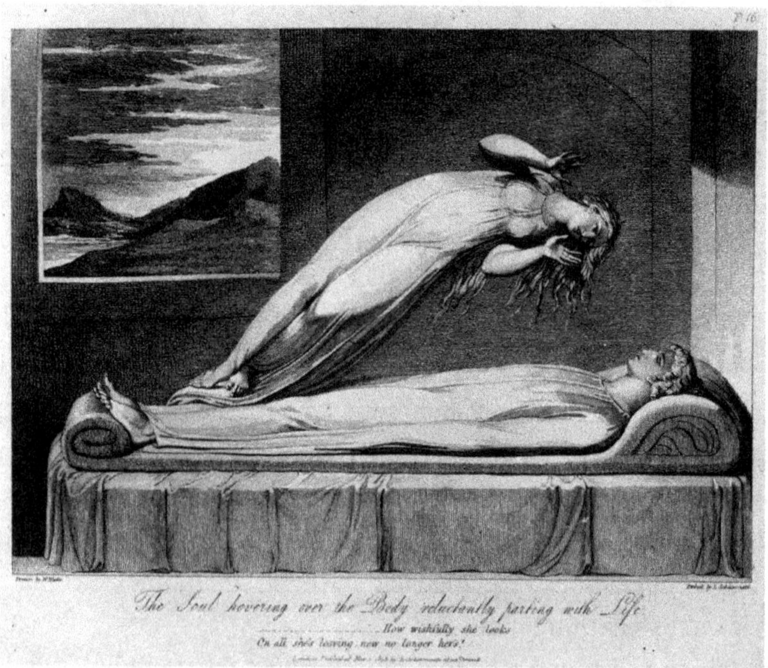

The Soul Leaving the Body, 1808, by Luigi Schiavonetti (†1810).
Wikimedia Commons: Public Domain

Many individuals describe a moment in which they shed their physical form, as if removing a coat, yet retain their full sense of self. From a vantage point above, they can observe their physical body—sometimes lifeless—and perceive the events around them with astonishing clarity. In medical settings such as operating rooms, physicians have verified cases where individuals could accurately describe conversations or procedures during a period when they were clinically dead. Nearly **90%** of those who report NDEs include an Out-of-Body-Experience.

2. Journey Through a Tunnel to a Heavenly Space

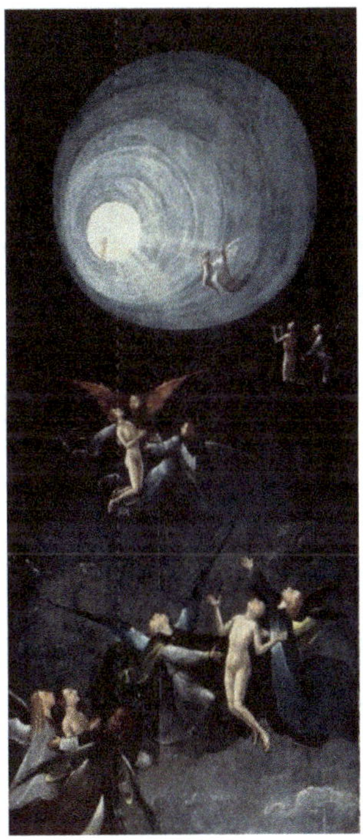

The Ascent of the Blessed, (1504) by Hieronymus Bosch (1450-1516). Depicts angels helping human souls towards heaven. Wikimedia Commons, Public Domain.

In NDE, this stage is often described as traveling through a dark tunnel toward a radiant light. Individuals of all religious backgrounds—even agnostics—report entering a realm of indescribable beauty and profound peace. There is a deep sense of **being loved unconditionally, without judgment**. While most describe this as a positive experience, a few encounter loneliness or fear perhaps due to the unfamiliar nature of the experience.

3. Life Review

In what feels like a brief moment in time, individuals report reviewing their entire life in extraordinary detail. This review is not passive; it is often experienced emotionally and relationally—feeling what others felt during one's own actions. Remarkably, even when unconscious for only minutes, many return able to speak for hours about this experience.

4. Timelessness and Connection

In the realm of the NDE, **time and distance seem to dissolve**. Individuals often feel a deep sense of connection to other people and even to all of creation. This awareness suggests a spiritual or quantum entanglement, where one's life is woven into a vast, interconnected web of being.

5. Meeting Deceased Loved Ones

Many describe **encounters with deceased relatives**. Communication in these moments often occurs through thought or inner knowing rather than words. These encounters feel real—deep, comforting, and personal—reinforcing the idea that consciousness may transcend death.

6. Encounter with a Divine Presence

Some NDE's report meeting a spiritual or divine figure or simply "the Light." Thus, the meeting appears influenced by one's particular religious tradition. NDEs communicate with the spiritual figure not verbally but mind to mind, or consciousness to consciousness.

7. Conscious Return to the Body

Re-entry into the body is often described as abrupt, sometimes entering through the top of the head. After returning, individuals are acutely aware of the limitations and pain of the physical body, and many report a sense of confinement compared to the freedom they just experienced.

8. Transformation and the Absence of Fear

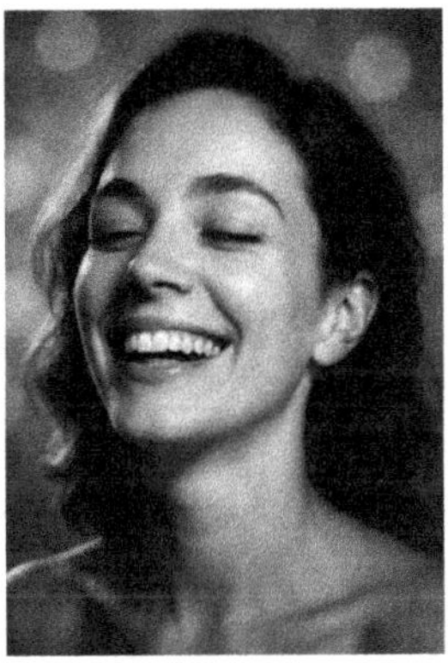

AI depicting profound peace and lack of fear following NDE

Upon re-entering their body, perhaps the most consistent aftereffect of an NDE is a **profound absence of the fear of death**. Many return with a renewed sense of purpose, a deeper capacity for love, and a heightened awareness of the interconnectedness of all life. Grudges, hatred, and resentment no longer make any sense. Life is seen through a spiritual lens.

Scientific Insights: Dr. Pim an Lommel

Dutch cardiologist Dr. Pim Van Lommel (2001) spent over 20 years researching NDEs. His extensive studies suggest that NDEs are not hallucinations or mere brain anomalies. In his work, Van Lommel states:

> The phenomenon of the NDE can no longer be scientifically ignored. The current materialist view of the relationship between consciousness and the brain seems too restricted. There are good reasons to assume that our consciousness, with the continuous experience of self, does not always coincide with the functioning of our brain. Enhanced or nonlocal consciousness, with unaltered self-identity, apparently can be experienced independently from the lifeless body.

Van Lommel's conclusion is that consciousness is not limited to the brain which indicates the brain functions more like the receiver of consciousness than its producer. Currently scientists assume consciousness is an epiphenomenon perhaps produced by the microtubules of the brain. In a later article, Van Lommel (2006) expresses the conclusion that consciousness can be experienced independently of brain function which may hopefully induce a change in the scientific paradigm in western medicine. He continues:

> Such understanding also fundamentally changes one's opinion about death, because of the almost unavoidable conclusion that at the time of physical death consciousness will continue to be experienced in another dimension, in an invisible and immaterial world, in which all past, present,

> and future is enclosed. Death is only the end of our physical aspects.

Because people with a NDE "almost" die, but do not die, the findings of studies on NDE cannot provide us the scientific proof as to whether consciousness does continue after death. What has been shown is that the NDE is experienced independently of brain function (Van Lommel's cardiac patients were declared dead) which indicates that without a functional body a human being can continue to have conscious experiences.

For many, there are more questions than answers, but we can also conclude that our daily consciousness is only a part of our whole consciousness.

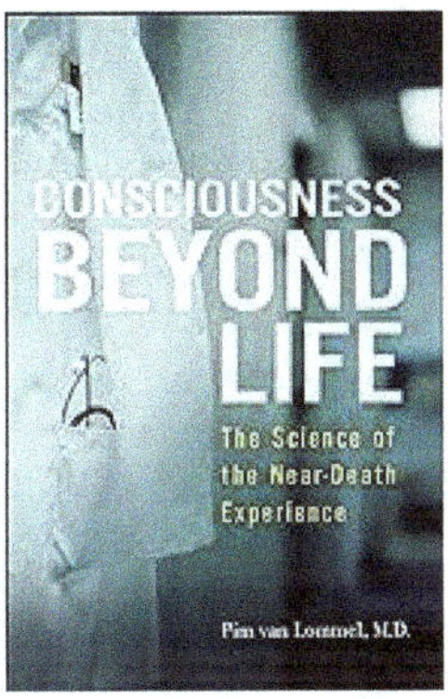

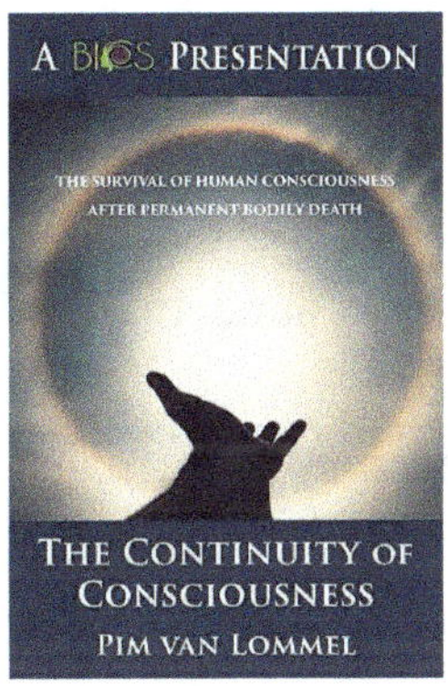

Van Lommel also believes there is an interconnection between informative fields of consciousness which explains the experience of enhanced awareness, dreams and visions, including visions experienced by a person near death and following death by loved ones. It is also when one feels connected to someone dying though separated by distance, and when able to communicate intuitively with deceased relatives at the time of death or afterwards.

This "enhanced" consciousness is believed to be due to the existence of universal fields of information where all knowledge, wisdom, and unconditional love are present and available. These fields of consciousness are believed to be stored in a dimension beyond our time and space, with universal interconnectedness. Van Lommel says one could call this our Higher consciousness, Divine consciousness, or Cosmic consciousness.

Evin Laszlo and Consciousness

Philosopher and scientist, Ervin Laszlo (2004) writes about the informational fields of consciousness where holographic memory is said to reside. The concept of an Information field is drawn from ancient Eastern spiritual traditions, called the Akashic Field, to describe a cosmic field containing all the information and knowledge about everyone and everything that has ever existed or ever will. It's often said this universal record of events, thoughts, and feelings is accessible to those who are gifted to make a connection because information in this field is said to be available indefinitely. Some believe this Information field is, in fact, the quantum plenum field of physics—thereby connecting spiritual concepts with scientific discoveries.

When a loved one dies, many communicate with their deceased loved one, not verbally, but intuitively—making a mental consciousness-to-consciousness connection—thereby affirming that human consciousness continues to exist after death. Only the body is left behind.

Dr. Van Lommel's and Ervin Laszlo's research challenges traditional scientific paradigms and opens the door to a more expansive view of life, death, and the soul.

Concluding Comments

Near-Death Experiences offer a powerful testament to the resilience and mystery of the human life. NDEs transcend cultural, religious, and scientific boundaries and offer a unifying vision of hope, love, and life beyond death. For those who have had them, **the experience is more real than real**—a glimpse of eternity through the window of dying. As we continue into Chapter 23, we will explore how the central theme of so many NDEs is not merely an emotion but the very foundation of reality. In the end, perhaps what binds us to one another and to the divine is the same force that awaits us in eternity.

Before moving to the next chapter, you may wish to ponder with the meaning of the Near-Death Experience.

- *Does NDE give you a glimpse of what we can anticipate in life after death?*
- *Any thoughts about Dr. Von Lommel's report from treating individuals who died of heart attack and had an out-of-body, Near-Death Experience?*
- *Have you communicated with a loved one after their death? If so, what was that like?*
- *Do you know someone who has communicated with their loved one after death?*

Chapter 23—Exploring Life After Death—Diverse Perspectives

As we approach the conclusion of Part IV, we broaden our view to explore the many perspectives that humanity has offered on one of life's most enduring mysteries: **What happens after we die?** Across time, cultures, and spiritual traditions, people have sought to understand the fate of the soul, the possibility of an afterlife, and the moral and metaphysical consequences of how we live. Many books have been written looking at the science of the Near-Death Experience.

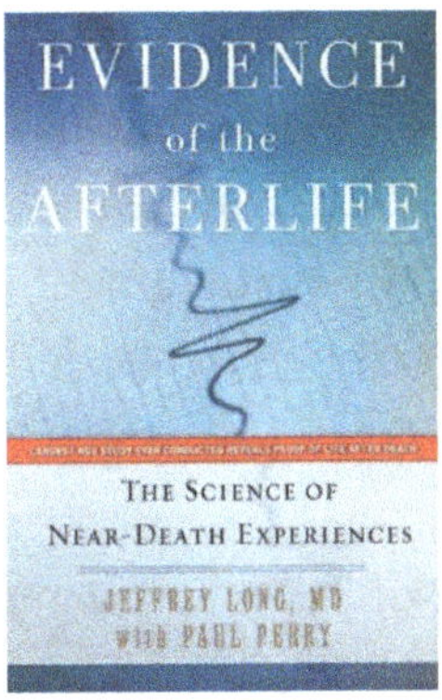

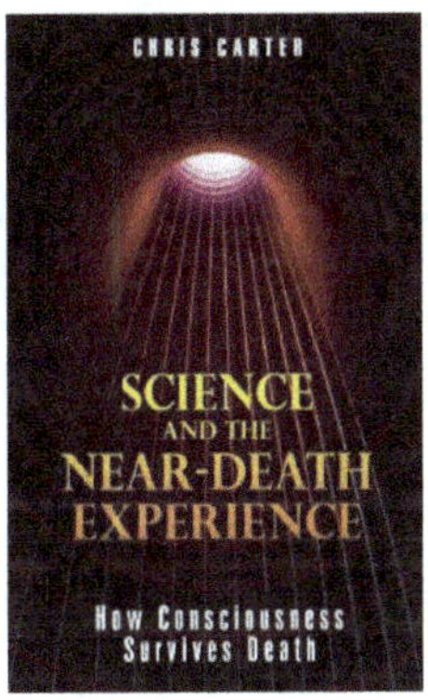

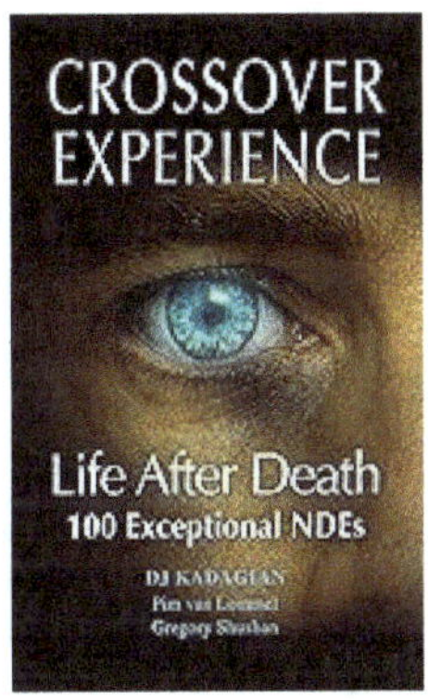

Americans Believe in the Afterlife

A 2021 survey by the Pew Research Center revealed 83% of Americans believe in an afterlife, with most believing in either heaven, hell, or both. Only 17% did not believe in life after death. 92% of self-professed Christians believe in heaven and 79% believe in hell. The number who believe in hell is highest among Evangelical Christians (91%). But to no surprise, there was disagreement as to who gets into heaven—30% believed there was only one path to heaven—

through the "one true faith"—theirs, of course. But many are open-minded about this. A majority said believers of "many religions" can gain eternal life. Interestingly, even theologians disagree—some hold to a "narrow gate" to heaven while others believed in "universal salvation," where everyone goes to heaven.

Perspectives from World Religions

This chapter surveys **Judeo-Christian, Eastern religious, and philosophical** perspectives on life after death. Though differing in language and imagery, many of these traditions reflect a shared yearning: that life does not end at death but is transformed.

Judaism

In Jewish tradition, beliefs about life after death have evolved through centuries of sacred reflection. In early Judaism, the concept of the afterlife was less defined, often referring to *Sheol*, the realm of the dead. Over time, ideas of bodily resurrection, divine judgment, and a more positive afterlife have evolved for many who embrace Judaism.

Christianity

Central to Christian belief is the resurrection of Jesus, viewed as the first fruits of a new creation, promising believers that death is not the end but the passage into eternal life. Heaven is portrayed as union with God, a realm of peace, joy, and love. Hell, by contrast, represents separation from God, sometimes metaphorically and sometimes interpreted literally. Salvation, in Christian theology, is understood to come through faith—trusting in God's grace through Jesus Christ—though many also emphasize the importance of good works, moral living, and love for others as expressions of that faith.

The Apostle Paul writes in 1 Corinthians 15:52: "The dead will be raised imperishable, and we shall be changed." This reflects the Christian hope of **transformation**—a continuation of life in a glorified form with God and all the heavenly host from every tribe and kindred on earth.

Eastern Religious Perspectives

In contrast to the linear view of life and afterlife in the West, Eastern religions often present a cyclical view of existence. In Hinduism, the soul *(Atman)* is eternal and passes through many lifetimes via **reincarnation**. One's actions in this life, known as **karma**, determine the circumstances of future lives. The ultimate goal is moksha, liberation from the cycle of rebirth and reunion with the divine (Brahman).

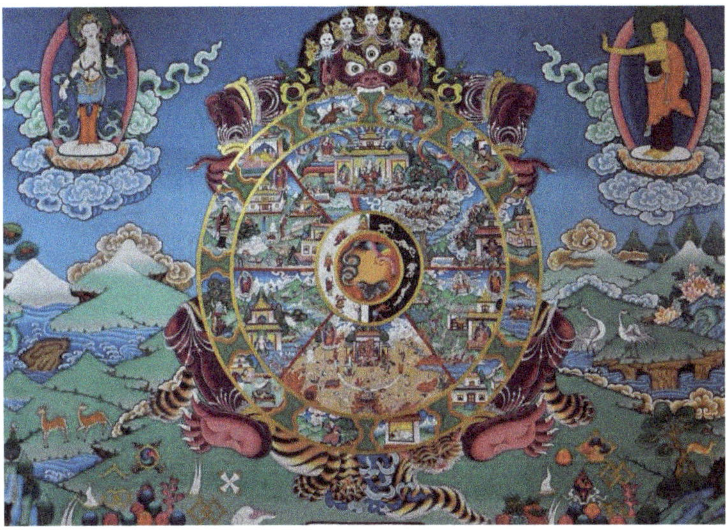

Buddhist *'Wheel Of Life'*—depicts the continuous cycle of existence from birth, death, and rebirth, influenced by karma where good and bad actions lead to different realms of rebirth. There are six realms of rebirth depicted around the wheel—including hell (at bottom), hungry ghosts, animals, humans, demi-gods, and God's realm. The path to liberation is through understanding and ethical actions. Author is Prof Ranga Sai (2013).

Buddhism, through the framework of rebirth and karma, emphasizes the impermanence of all things and the absence of a permanent self. Depicted above is the *Six Realms of the Wheel of Life* representing the different states of existence that beings can be reborn into, based on their karma and actions in previous lives. The cycle of reincarnation and rebirths continues until reaching the goal, which is Nirvana, the cessation of suffering and liberation from the cycle of samsara. This is achieved through the cultivation of wisdom, ethical living, and meditation.

Taoism. Here the focus less on specific destinations after death and more on living in harmony with the Tao, the flow of the universe. Death is seen as a return to the source—a transformation, not an ending.

These traditions challenge us to see life after death not only as reward or punishment, but as a continuation of spiritual evolution—a journey of the soul toward unity, wisdom, and freedom (Kripal et al., 2024).

Philosophical Perspectives

Philosophers, too, have long wrestled with the question of what, if anything, comes after death. **Plato** proposed that the soul is immortal and continues its journey after the body dies. In his dialogues, he describes death as the soul's release from the prison of the body.

Descartes advanced the mind-body dualism theory, suggesting that mind (or soul) and body are separate substances. This opens the door to imagining consciousness continuing without the physical form. Yet materialist philosophers, from **David Hume** to modern secular thinkers, argue that consciousness is a byproduct of the brain and ceases when the brain dies.

Contemporary debates center around the **mind-body problem**—how the subjective experience of mind arises from the physical processes of the brain. Some neuroscientists now consider the possibility of **consciousness as nonlocal**—a view that consciousness is not a by-product of the brain. This view supported by research into near-death experiences, quantum theory, and transpersonal psychology as mentioned in previous chapters.

While philosophy may not provide definitive answers, it enriches the discussion by reminding us of the depth and diversity of human reasoning—and our persistent intuition that death is not the end of the story.

Post-Science and Life After Death

Harvard educated and Director of the Human Energy Systems Laboratory in the Department of Neurology at the University of Arizona, Gary E. Schwartz, Ph.D., is a prominent voice in advancing post-materialist science. His research has centered on exploring consciousness, spirituality, and examining apparently nonrandom patterns of events in real life as valid and meaningful evidence of the presence of higher spiritual forces.

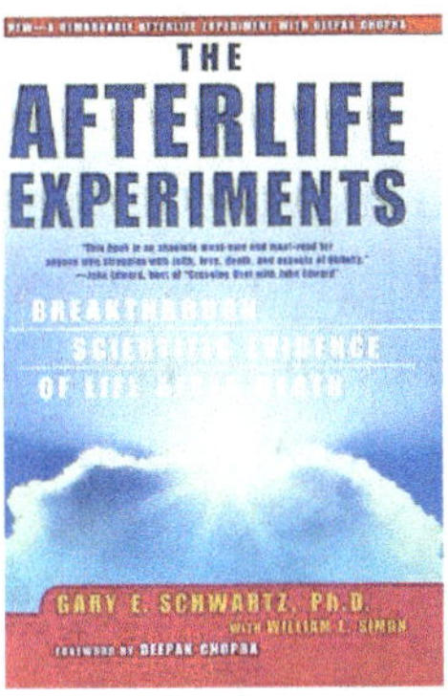

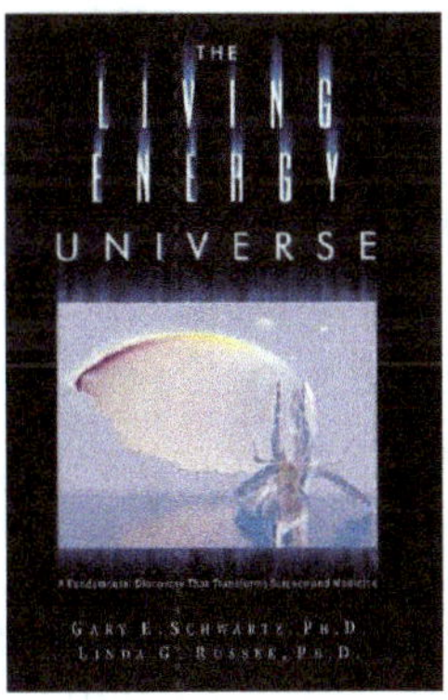

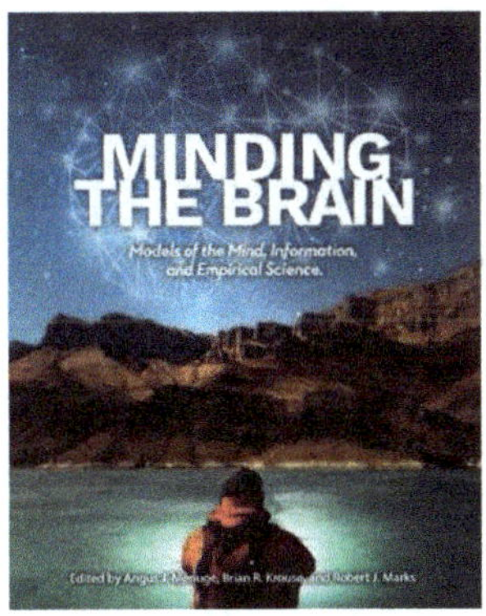

In his book, *The Afterlife Experiments* (2002), Schwartz, together with researcher Linda Russek, Ph.D., worked with professional mediums to investigate whether there is life after death. The book provides examples of precognition and observations by mediums. Information obtained from the deceased through the mediums led

Schwartz to say, "The data appear to be as valid, convincing, and living as the mediums, sitters, skeptics, and scientists themselves." Scientific reports in the Appendix of his book are used to support the scientific foundation for Schwartz and Russek's work, as does their earlier book *The Living Energy Universe* (1999).

Death at the Movies

Bassett (2014) looked at the attitudes of individuals about immortality and the Afterlife in selected movies. He says,

> Afterlife beliefs can simultaneously assuage fears of personal extinction and magnify anxieties about the specifics of post-death experience, identity, and relationships. Immortality is appealing because it quells anxiety about death; however, examination of whether finite human psychology would, if faced with eternity, be able to preserve identity while avoiding monotony raises doubts about the feasibility and desirability of eternal life, as certain films illustrate.

Bassett says that analysis of selected movies with after-life themes can offer valuable insight into viewers' interest in and concerns about eternity. What movies can do is enable the individual to ask whether the values that uphold our theological positions about death are defensible just because they happen to have been around in human cultures for centuries.

Films about the afterlife can mitigate the fears some hold about the afterlife by offering the idea that eternity will be a pleasant experience. At the same time depictions of the afterlife in film can raise concern about whether it will be possible to maintain an eternally pleasant existence for all eternity. This leads some to say they do not want to live forever. For these reasons, viewer reactions to afterlife films is often ambivalent.

Among the movies Bassett discusses are *Star Wars III: Revenge of the Sith* (2005) where Anakin is plagued with guilt over his failure to prevent the death of his mother portraying death as an essential aspect of being human and the anxiety we have concerning our death, as well as denial of death by the belief we can conquer it.

Conversely, in *Star Trek: Generations* (1994) the scientist Soren, who is obsessed with the fear of death and seeks to achieve immortality by entering a cosmic energy field, called Nexus, where time does not exist. In attempting to stop Soren, Captain Picard argues that it is our mortality that defines us as being human. Turns out, we learn Picard is also struggling with death because of his advancing age and the fact he has no children to carry on his legacy.

In his article, Bassett also mentions Stephen Cave (2012) who describes how our cognitive capacities give rise in humanity to contradictory attitudes about death which he calls "**the mortality paradox**." The paradox arises because, on-the-one-hand we are aware that all living things must die, and on-the-other-hand we are unable to grasp that we will die. To avoid this distressing ambivalence, we convince ourselves we are **immortal**, immune to death. Death happens to others but will not happen to us. In other words, we are both certain all must die one day and yet in denial about our death. Cave explains this is why we develop stories to help make sense of this "**existential impasse**."

Death and Immortality in Books

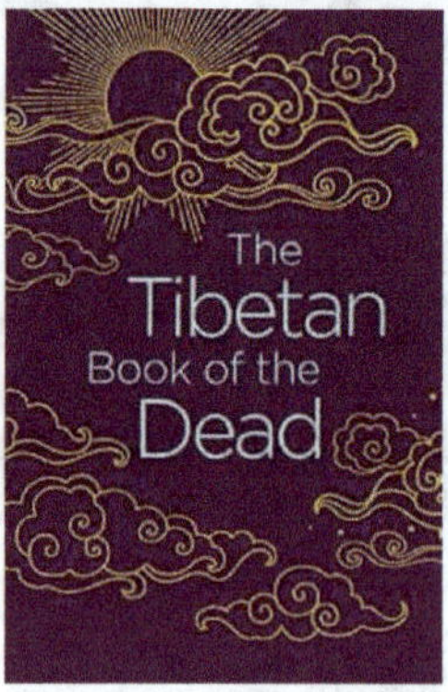

The Tibetan Book of the Dead—is a sacred Buddhist text used to guide the soul through the process of death, the intermediate state (bardo), and eventual rebirth or liberation.

The Tibetan Book of the Dead—well known to Tibetans as the *Bardo Thodol* ("Liberation Through Hearing in the Intermediate State")—teaches that consciousness continues after death and journeys through various stages, encountering peaceful and wrathful deities that are ultimately projections of one's own mind. The text is often read aloud to the dying (or recently deceased) to aid them in attaining to enlightenment and thereby escaping the cycle of reincarnation. The readings emphasize awareness, detachment, and the transformative power of realizing the true nature of reality—an illumined existence beyond ego and illusion.

This sacred text reveals a core Tibetan Buddhist belief—that death is not an end, but a passage into a profound state of potential awakening. In this vision, the soul enters the bardo, a luminous realm between death and rebirth, where the ultimate destiny of the soul is shaped not by judgment, but by consciousness itself. Eternity, then, is not a distant afterlife but an ever-present dimension that we awaken to through awareness. As modern science begins to explore consciousness beyond the brain, the ancient voice of The Tibetan Book of the Dead points forward: death is not darkness, but the unveiling of a deeper light—one that the awakened mind can recognize as its true nature.

Tuesdays With Morrie, by Mitch Albom, is a deeply moving memoir that chronicles the author's weekly visits with his former college professor, Morrie Schwartz, during the final months of Morrie's life. As Morrie slowly succumbs to ALS (Lou Gehrig's disease), he shares profound life lessons on love, work, aging, forgiveness, and ultimately, death. Framed as a series of "last visits," the book transforms Morrie's dying into wisdom for how to live meaningfully. With warmth, humor, and emotional honesty, Morrie confronts death not with fear but with acceptance and gratitude, seeing it as a natural part of life. The book's central message is that embracing our mortality can awaken us to what truly matters—compassion, connection, and living with purpose. In the book we read: "Death ends a life, not a relationship."

This simple statement embodies profound insight—"Death ends a life, not a relationship"—and offers a lens through which to view the eternal. While the physical body may perish, the love we share, the meaning we create, and the spiritual essence we carry do not vanish. In many traditions, eternity is not merely a span of unending time but a dimension where presence, connection, and consciousness transcend physical form. Morrie's wisdom invites us to see death not as a wall, but as transformation—a doorway rather than an end. Just as quantum physics suggests particles remain entangled across space and time, so too might our souls remain bound by love, beyond the veil of mortality.

The Last Lecture is a heartfelt and inspiring memoir by Dr. Randy Pausch, a computer science professor at Carnegie Mellon University, written after his diagnosis with terminal pancreatic cancer. With only months to live, Pausch chose to deliver a "last lecture" not about dying but about living well. Titled *"Really Achieving Your Childhood Dreams,"* the talk—later turned into this bestselling book—offers lessons on perseverance, imagination, humility, and love. With warmth and wit, Pausch reflects on his life's joys and regrets, aiming to leave a legacy not only for his students and readers, but especially for his young children. *The Last Lecture* can be viewed on YouTube and is a celebration showing how one's spirit can transcend the limits of time.

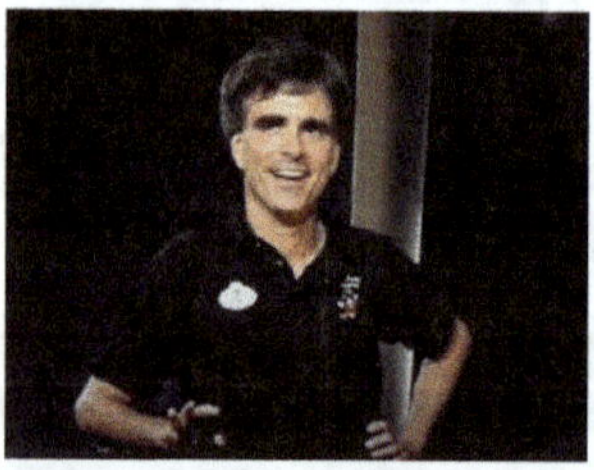

Carnegie Mellon Professor Randy Pausch (Oct. 23, 1960 - July 25, 2008) gave his last lecture at the university Sept. 18, 2007. Public Domain, YouTube.com: "Randy Pausch's Last Lecture." https://www.youtube.com/watch?v=ji5_MqicxSo

Randy Pausch's final reflections are a modern echo of timeless spiritual truths—that a life filled with purpose, love, and integrity leaves behind something unforgettable. Though his physical life was ending, his message reached millions, rippling outward in ways that far outlasted his body. In this sense, *The Last Lecture* is not simply a farewell—it is a testament to the eternal nature of wisdom and love. Just as sacred texts and rituals carry meaning across generations, Pausch's words remind us that eternity is not confined to the heavens but is etched into the hearts and memories of those we touch. His story affirms that living consciously in the face of death can awaken us to the eternal present and the enduring impact of a well-lived life.

Concluding Comments

Across spiritual and philosophical traditions, the afterlife is imagined in many forms: heaven and hell, reincarnation and liberation, eternal presence or ceaseless transformation. Whether seen as a realm of reward, a cycle of refinement, or a return to the divine source, life after death remains one of the deepest longings and inquiries of the human spirit.

In the final chapter of Part IV, we will return to the central force that permeates all these perspectives—Love. What if love is not only our guide in this life, but the very energy that receives us in the next? Join me as we reflect on **Love as the Final Word**.

Before we move on, consider these questions thoughtfully:

- *83% of Americans believe in an afterlife, with most believing in either heaven, hell, or both. What are your thoughts about life after death?*
- *In our survey of world religions, what do you make of their similarities concerning the afterlife?*
- *Do the different views about the afterlife cause you concern?*
- *Can you recall a movie about life after death? How did you respond to it?*
- *Any thoughts about "Tuesdays with Morie" and Randy Pausch "Last Lecture?"*

Chapter 24—Love as the Final Word

We began with mystery, and we end with love.

This book has been a journey looking at steps of reconciliation, of how we find the place of unity in the face of separation and division. In particular, this has been a deep consideration of **science and spirituality**, of the physical and the unseen, of the measurable and the miraculous, which together embrace the whole of reality that we experience as human beings on planet Earth. We have walked through the architecture of belief, stood in awe before the miracle of existence, glimpsed the workings of quantum mechanics, and dared to imagine what lies beyond death. Along the way, we have returned again and again to one recurring theme: that consciousness is not isolated, but shared; that reality is not random, but relational; and that, at the heart of it all, **there is Love**.

Love is not just an emotion. It is a force—a field, a vibration, a binding energy. In the quantum realm, every sub-atomic particle vibrates with the rhythm of the universe, and entangled particles communicate across vast distances instantly, as though they were never truly apart. Is this not a mirror of our own spiritual entanglement with one another and with the divine? If the universe is, at its core, a web of interconnected energy and information, then love is the thread that holds the web together.

Three Simple Yet Meaningful Stories

Recently, in a meeting of our bereavement support group, a member shared that the day before a small bird had crashed into a window at her office and the bird flew for a moment, then landed in the middle of a street. She didn't want a car or truck to run over the little bird, so she gathered it up and that is when she realized it was dead. Interestingly, this whole time there were about ten birds swirling about and appeared to be observing what was happening to the little bird. Not wanting to throw the bird in the trash, she and her co-workers put the little bird in a box, and they held a memorial service for the bird before its burial. When they finished, amazingly the other ten birds departed.

After this story, several in the group began telling their stories. One shared that when she was a child, a goldfish died and that she and friends held a service for the dead goldfish. She and her friends even covered their heads in reverence. She said when her grandfather saw what was taking place he was deeply touched and complimented the children.

Yet another shared that her husband had recently found a dead fly that was stuck on the outside of a windowpane in their home. He took a picture of the fly on the windowpane and named it, "A lesser life." He said he did not mean to denigrate the life of the fly by calling it a "lesser life." Instead, he wanted to affirm that the fly had been alive and that its life had meaning, though in a very different way from a human life.

These stories are a reminder that throughout our life, and even as a child, we experience encounters with death, and it is often with an awareness that an animal or a butterfly or goldfish is no longer alive. It is no longer able to swim or fly or play with others of its kind. No longer able to be with its mother, father, or siblings. And the fact we hold all life is reverent whether a dog or cat, goldfish or a fly, speaks volumes about how meaningful every life is, including our own life and that of those we love.

The Language of Universal Consciousness—Love

Love can be understood as the gentle whisper of the Absolute One who brought forth light from darkness, order from chaos, and life from stillness. It is what draws us toward each other in compassion, what lifts us beyond ourselves in sacrifice, and what anchors our belief that death is not the end.

In our exploration of **quantum physics**, we have seen how the smallest units of matter are not truly solid, but rather are **fields of probability**, blinking in and out of existence at the speed of light. We have seen that information, not matter, may be the most fundamental reality—an insight that harmonizes with ancient spiritual wisdom. In the language of faith, this information is divine thought; it is the Word made flesh. In the language of science, it is the structure beneath structure, the music beyond sub-atomic particles.

To bring together science and spirituality is not to blend one into the other, but to let each illuminate the other. **Science explains how; spirituality asks why**. Science gives us laws; spirituality gives us meaning. And in the union of the two, we come to see that the universe is not a machine, but a mystery. A sacred, loving mystery.

What we have called God may well be the very fabric of consciousness that undergirds all things—the Infinite Mind, the Ground of Being, the Intelligent Light, the Source. In this vision, humans are not separate sparks of light doomed to flicker and vanish. We are waves upon an eternal sea. We rise, we fall, but we are never lost.

Near-death experiences affirm this truth. People return with the conviction that the most important reality is not what we have done, but **how we have loved**. And they bring back a clarity that all is connected, that consciousness continues, and that love is the source and our destination.

Love and World Religions

All the world's religions—when stripped of their cultural trappings—point toward this truth. The Hebrew Scriptures proclaim that God's steadfast love endures forever. Judeo-Christianity proclaims God is love. Islam teaches Allah is love. The Upanishads whisper that the self and the divine are one. The Buddha taught compassion for all sentient beings. Love is the universal doctrine, the cosmic signature.

Christian Psychologist, Margaret G. Alter (1994) has written:

> We embody an untarnished holiness, and by God's design nothing we do can change that fact. We are created in the image of God and chosen for friendship with God. We are forgiven for the isolating, perfectionistic burdens we undertake in our futile efforts to become God, to be ultimately safe. The call to friendship is a call to community, a call to love one another and to care for our world. In the biblical tradition, we are a servant people called that the nations of the world might bless themselves.

Co-creator with the Divine

Although it may be surprising to say we are co-creators with The Source, the creator of the universe, with God, but the fact is every decision and action we take is either in alignment with the Will of God or it is contrary to divine will. This means **we are co-creators**—for good or for not so good—and this is true whether or not we acknowledge it is taking place. Co-creation implies that our choices, actions, and behavior are intentional, not arbitrary or ambivalent—that we intend to flow with the divine will for our lives and within our sphere of influence.

To explain further the idea of being co-creator with God, Manuel G. Doncel, S. J., (2004), Professor emeritus of fundamental theology and of theoretical particle physics at Universitat Autònoma de Barcelona, says:

> I distinguish between the limitations and responsibilities of the human being as a created agent and the possibilities and ideals as a co-creator, created in the image of God. In what

> follows I develop the deep idea of the Creator's kenosis (self-emptying), which constitutes the very root of God's love principle and should then be personally and socially reenacted by the created co-creators.

Fr. Doncel points out the Christian idea of **kenosis ("self-emptying")** is grounded in the New Testament understanding of the Incarnation of Jesus of Nazareth as expressed in Philippians 2:7 which speaks of Christ's life and death on the Cross, "he emptied himself, taking on the form of a slave, coming in human likeness." Doncel also says this points to the need to renew the concept of the nature of God from being one of absolute power to recognize God who is absolute love and kenosis being the principal characteristic of any love relation. Doncel says, "the Creator's kenosis appears to us as **love's endeavor**, a work of love." And, God's love is universal and applicable to all people, the good and the bad.

Co-Creators with God

The Book of Genesis in the Bible says human beings are created in the image of God. This means we are intended to imitate God and are given the freedom and responsibility to choose to flow within the divine will, which is **self-emptying love**. However, Fr. Doncel says the intent of God is for created persons to "work beside the Creator as his craftsman." Although intended by God to be co-creators of the divine will, we experience our weakness and self-serving human nature; and we experience the richness of human situation as we become consciously aware of our call to be the Creator's instrument to bring about wholeness and well-being in every aspect of the world. And, as the life of Jesus Christ revealed, the way is Kenosis, **self-emptying, genuine love**.

According to the love principal, we are called to love our neighbor and Fr. Doncel says with the internet and global communication, all nations and people of the planet, regardless of race, culture, or religious belief—all are our neighbors.

Our Sphere of Influence

As co-creators with God, we are to exercise our self-emptying love for all people and all of creation within our **sphere of Influence**. Our sphere of influence is usually much larger than we acknowledge. Many will say "I have no influence" although that is not true. Every word spoken, every choice made, and every action taken impact others—especially one's spouse, children, close friends and peer group. Over time many are placed in a position of leadership that directly influences others either at work or in their religious community. We influence others through the words we say to them and through what we write in emails and over the internet, in notes and letters, or by a book we share with others because it touched us deeply. All these acts influence others, including all that which we create with our hands and heart. A few among us are elected to public office and their actions, or inaction, will impact countless individuals they will never know personally.

Ponder your sphere of influence with gratitude and a measure of humility.

As co-creators with the divine, we are centered in the ultimate consciousness of the universe, God. Our thoughts and words matter. Words express our beliefs, and beliefs inform our choices.

An important question to ask is, **"Am I a co-creator with God?"** As hard as it may be to answer in the affirmative, professing this reality can be transformative for you and others. The belief and awareness that we are a co-creator with God gives ultimate meaning and purpose to one's life.

How do we co-create with God? With love. Every act of love expressed is in alignment with the will of God. We are not alone. We each have a sphere of influence. Value it. Cultivate it.

Concluding Comments

As this book closes, we return to the beginning in reverence. In the Preface I said that although the long-awaited Theory of Everything (TOE) in physics refers to the union of classical and quantum physics, for me when science and spirituality come together, they inform what could become an ultimate, unified, singular, all-encompassing, coherent Theory of Reality (TOR) under the over-arching love of God. Even beyond a theory of reality, the deepest beliefs and discoveries of physics and the oldest insights of mysticism converge here: Love is not an afterthought. It is the final word.

As we each approach the end of our life, the final words that will be said over us will likely come from the faith tradition that has spoken love to our heart—be they words from the Tibetan Book of the Dead if we are Buddhist, or the service of *Levayah* if we are Jewish. The word *Levayah* means "escorting" and signifies the act of accompanying the deceased to their final resting place. Being a life-long Christian, the words said for me will come from The Burial of the Dead service found in the Episcopal Church's Book of Common Prayer (p. 491), which reads:

> I am Resurrection and I am life, says the Lord.
> Whoever has faith in me shall have life, even though he die.
> And everyone who has life and has committed himself to me
> Shall not die for ever.
>
> As for me, I know that my Redeemer lives
> And that at the last he will stand upon the earth.
> After my awaking, he will raise me up;
> and in my body I shall see God.
> I myself shall see, and my eyes behold him
> who is my friend, and not as a stranger.

For none of us has life in himself,
and none becomes his own master when he dies.
For if we have life, we are alive in the Lord,
and if we die, we die in the Lord.
So, then, whether we live or die,
We are the Lord's possession.
Happy from now on are those who die in the Lord!

I will also ask a passage to be read for me from Revelation 21:4-7

"Now the dwelling of God is among mortals, and He will dwell with them. They will be his people, and God himself will be with them and be their God. He will wipe away every tear from their eyes. There will be no more death or morning or crying or pain, for the first order of things has passed away.

Then, he who was seated on the throne said, "I am making all things new!" Then he said to me: "Write this down, for these words are trustworthy and true." He said to me, "It is done! I am the Alpha and Omega, the beginning and the end. To those who are thirsty I will give to drink freely from the spring of the water of life. Those who overcome will inherit all this, and I will be their God, and they will be my children.

May love be my final word and your final word as well. To live in love is to live in alignment with the quantum soul, with divine consciousness, with eternity itself. To speak love, to act in love, and to choose love—this is our highest calling, and our truest destiny.

May this love guide you, hold you, and awaken you. In this great unfolding universe, you are not alone. You are known. You are part of the Whole. And the Whole is love. Let there be light.

Final questions to prayerfully and thoughtfully consider:

- *How did you respond to the three simple stories of how throughout our life we learn about death by our encounters with the death of animals, birds, and even a fly?*
- *Have you ever thought of yourself as a Co-creator with God?*
- *Ever thought about your sphere of influence? What responsibilities does this imply?*
- *Have you thought about your own death? Planned your own funeral service?*

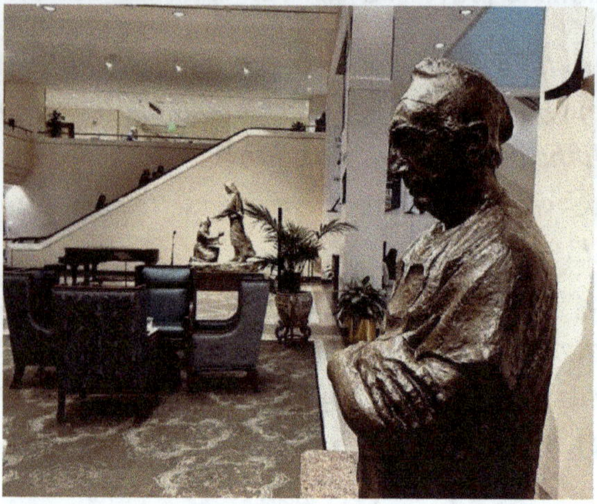

There are two statues in the lobby of Houston Methodist Hospital which express what this book is all about.

Dr. Michael DeBakey (medical science) and Jesus' healing touch (spirituality)

Notice the spiritual dimension is "distant"—easily overlooked—but is ever present.

Science and Spirituality are united and serve together

Photography by Fr. John K Graham

Afterword

My Current Beliefs on Life, Science, Faith, and Life After Death

Creation and The Source

The universe exists because consciousness—Divine Intelligence—called it into being. Whether we name this our Higher Power, God, The Absolute One, "Ultimate Reality," "The Source," "Universal Mind," or "Ultimate Consciousness," we speak of the same boundless Mystery. Thirteen-point-eight billion years ago, this Mystery breathed existence into being at what is called the Big Bang—or, I prefer saying that creation took place when God, Universal Mind, breathed out the Big Breath!

The Source, God, has been revealed to all people, in every age, across every culture and tradition. Thus, the manifold religions of the world—each pointing, however partially, to the same eternal Mystery. Whether known as Allah, Krishna, Yahweh, Brahman, God, Jesus, or the Great Spirit, the Divine has always made itself known.

God is not an old man in the sky, as Renaissance art might suggest, but a spiritual Presence—pure, intelligent, aware—permeating all that is. God is both transcendent, beyond time and space, and immanent, intimately present in the unfolding of every moment, from the orbit of distant stars to the breath in our lungs.

As thousands of new planets are discovered in our galaxy, we begin to glimpse just how vast God's awareness must be. Every atom, every creature, every unknown world is known to The Source. As a mother with her child, God is not passive but deeply participatory—a presence that receives, holds, and responds to all things everywhere. In other words, God is relational.

Reality, as I understand it, unfolds in three interwoven levels: the material, the quantum, and the virtual. The material is our daily world of solidity and time. Deep within, the quantum level is a realm of mystery, possibility and potentiality—where particles blink in and out of existence, and an act of interaction (or a spoken word) can affirm or change outcomes. Deeper still, lies the virtual level, the ground of being—pure consciousness, the informational field from which all things emerge. These levels flow into one another like the currents of a stream: the virtual that births, and the quantum that manifests the material. When we begin to grasp these interpenetrating layers, we start to perceive a scaffolding for the miraculous.

From the moment of creation, the Source established the laws of physics. These laws are not broken by miracles; rather, the miraculous is an alignment—astonishing and lawful—a gesture pointing toward a greater Intelligence and Presence, the Sacred, God.

Science and Faith: Partners in Truth

The era of materialism's dominance is fading. Science and religion, often seen as adversaries, are in truth twin pursuits of the same mystery. Both seek understanding. Both depend on awareness. Both seek to bless humanity and creation. And both, at their best, point to something greater than themselves.

Why do scientists remain silent on the spiritual implications of their work? Perhaps because truth, though simple and radical, is considered dangerous. Many scientists realistically fear ridicule or dismissal. Their field is physics, not metaphysics, they may say—and rightly so, unless they have awakened to the divine Mystery. Religion, too, has often failed to speak this truth—not out of malice, but perhaps fear. Fear of losing power, fear of losing the certainty of their traditions, or perhaps simply a lack of understanding of the deep connection between the quantum world and the spiritual one.

While I have been a life-long Christian and join others in affirming the words of the Nicene Creed every Sunday, I understand all world's religions, including Christianity, at their best, point to the true Source, the eternal God. In our religious settings we gather with other men and women of faith to celebrate the mystery of God. This is good and can be life-giving. Yet, organized religion can also distract us from maintaining our connection with the Ultimate Reality. Spiritual practices, such as prayer, meditation, and contemplation that focus on the divine can help maintain that connection, as can walking in one's neighborhood with gratitude and love for the beauty of God's creation in a tree, in a flower, or in a bird that flies overhead. Energy cannot be destroyed—it only changes form. So too with consciousness. When the body dies, the egoic personality dissolves, but the essence remains. Our thoughts, emotions, and experiences are preserved in the quantum field. This is why we sense déjà vu, premonitions, and the presence of the departed. These are echoes of that eternal field.

Suffering is not meaningless. In Buddhism, it is a school. Just as muscles grow under strain, the soul is strengthened through adversity. Every loss, every trial is part of a curriculum designed for growth. One day, we will understand what may now seem senseless—and we will know we were never alone.

Unity or Chaos: The Choice Before Us

All spiritual paths, at their core, point toward unity, The Source. And yet, in our time, humanity drifts toward division. Our technology races ahead, while our spiritual development lags. We forget that we are one body, one breath, one family. We see enemies instead of mirrors. This is a grave danger in a nuclear age. We must awaken to our oneness—or we risk our own extinction. As Dr. Martin Luther King, Jr. said, we face a choice: chaos or community.

The enemy is not another race, nation, or religion. Nor is science the enemy. The enemy is ignorance. And the only true weapon against ignorance is light—knowledge, wisdom, truth. But this truth cannot be imposed. It must be received. Each soul must awaken in its own time. What lies beyond death is not the primary question. The question is: how shall we live while alive? The answer is always the same: love.

The Soul Beyond the Laboratory

Science asks for proof—measurability and repeatability. But the deepest truths do not fit neatly into laboratories. With deep truth repeatability is not statistical but existential. They show up in every culture, every generation, in stories of near-death, past-life memory, and quantum mysteries that defy logic but not experience. Science may resist, but resistance is not proof. Every great scientific leap was once mocked or ignored. Quantum physics has already torn a hole in materialism: time is not fixed, space is not empty, and matter is not solid. All is energy. All is consciousness. All is interconnected. All is unity. Life is miraculous!

The true work before us is not to convince the skeptical, but to live as if we knew death was not the end. If every person believed that thoughts, words, and deeds were eternal—preserved in the quantum field—our world would be awakened and transformed.

A Lifelong Search for What Is Real

I am, at heart, a seeker. Truth has never been, for me, found in government, religion, or science alone. Human institutions may point to the truth, but too often become idols—substitutes for The Source they claim to serve.

In my youth, I longed to understand: What is real? Why am I here? And, later in life, I wanted to know what matters for my wife, children, grandchildren, and for the world? Over time, I've discovered the hardest question of all is this: Who am I? Why do I do what I do, and fail to do what I know is right? St. Paul wrestled with the same question in Romans 7: "For the good I desire, I do not do, but the evil I hate, that I do."

The journey inward is the longest and most necessary one. I find joy in biology, in the brilliant intricacy of the cell. But science cannot answer the deeper question: What is the meaning of life?

We fear death because we do not want to lose what we know and love. Yet what awaits us is far greater than what we leave behind. Eternal life with God—filled with imagination, creativity, and divine love—this is the real promise. Awesome, indeed beyond what we can conceive or imagine.

My encounters with the Living God changed me. Such encounters are unforgettable. They become part of one's very being. A single encounter with The Source can illuminate a lifetime. Nothing—no scientific breakthrough, no worldly success—compares. Absolutely nothing.

What is true will endure. Love, kindness, memory, beauty—these go with us and before us.

So, live in search of Truth. Love courageously. And know: The Source, God, is always present.

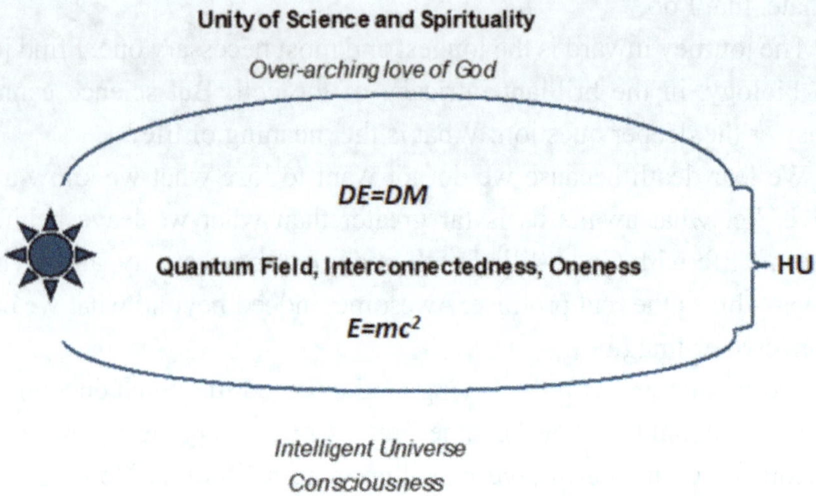

The above drawing depicts the union of science and spirituality under the overarching love of God. It begins on the left with the Big Bang (Big Breath) and in the center are symbols of physics: *DE=DM* representing Dark Energy and Dark Matter and below is Einstein's equation $E=mc^2$. In the middle is the interconnected Quantum Unified Field of sub-atomic particles of possibilities and probabilities which attests that at the quantum level there is only oneness for all things and all people. Below is depicted the Intelligent Universe and Universal Consciousness. To the right, HU, the holographic universe. This depicts the whole of reality, both science and spirituality.

Appendix—Four Encounters

After reading my book you may reasonably ask yourself: "Why should I listen to anything he has to say?"

That's a fair question.

It's important for you to discern whether there is authenticity and integrity when I speak of things spiritual. Are my words simply the product of a logical and reasoning mind, or do they arise from a heart that has been truly transformed by an encounter with the living God?

What follows are four stories from my life—moments I believe to be genuine encounters with the divine. If you find them implausible or unconvincing, I will understand. But if even one of these stories stirs something in you—if you find even a spark of resonance—then perhaps you'll want to walk with me even further. If that is true, at the end of these four encounters, you will find an opportunity for us to journey together into the mystery that lies ahead.

Encounter One: Story of Emptiness, Good Works, and the Divine

In this book I have shared my understanding of the biology of belief and belief's power to transform our lives. For that reason, I need to share is my own story of transformation.

At 35 years old, I had achieved everything I was told would bring fulfillment—a beautiful two-story English Tudor home in the best part of town, a thriving medical practice, a big car, a loving wife, and five wonderful children.

Yet inside, I was empty and began to wonder, *Is this all there is to life?* Though I had grown up in a Protestant church, memorized scripture as a boy, and still attended church services, I wasn't truly connected with God. That disconnect, I believe, was the root of my emptiness.

I explored everything I could to fill the void—I devoured books on Eastern religion, practiced yoga (I could even stand on my head with feet in the air), and chased meaning in all kinds of ideas. But nothing satisfied me.

One Sunday afternoon, I sat by our backyard swimming pool watching my children splash and laugh. And I thought, *My kids will grow up and one day feel what I feel—this same emptiness, the same lack of purpose.* At the time, I had been reading a book by the Humanist Society entitled Moral Essays on Contemporary Society.

The first half of the book, "The Reality of the World Today," argued that religious leaders had invented a God in their own image—meant to meet psychological needs. I thought, *Exactly, that's what I believe!* I turned eagerly to the second part of the book, entitled "The Good Life," hoping for some insight to fill the emptiness I felt. But it offered no true solace. It said: There is no God. We must make life meaningful ourselves—by making the world a better place to live.

I turned the book face-down in frustration. I thought, *They don't have the answers either.*

That was especially disheartening because for over a decade, I had been doing just that—trying to make the world better. I had even worked with prison inmates for a year, helping them put on a play that I wrote, *The Axion Experiments*—a story about the search for meaning, which ends with love as the ultimate truth.

The experience of putting on the play was electric. The inmates poured themselves into their roles. An individual produced impressive visuals by utilizing an overhead projector and paint. Others built the stage, prepared chairs for guests. We invited the public. Standing ovations followed every performance. *The Shreveport Times* ran a two-page spread on the play, quoting one inmate: "This is the most constructive thing I've ever done."

We performed several times at Shreveport's Centenary College, again to standing ovations. Then in Dallas, I treated the men to a fine dinner atop the Southland Life Tower. The next day, we performed at a large Methodist church to another standing ovation. I thought we were Broadway-bound.

But back home, reality hit. The inmates, released on good behavior, began drifting. My wife and I took one into our home, but we didn't have room for them all. One Sunday morning I picked up the paper and saw the headline: **GOVERNOR RAIDS COLUMBIA PARK**. Every one of the men I had worked with was listed. Arrested. Back in prison.

I was heartbroken. I loved those men. And the play that had symbolized hope and purpose was shattered. I had tried to do good, and it hadn't been enough. *I must not truly understand love, I thought. I'm still empty.*

And then, something remarkable happened.

That very Sunday afternoon, sitting by the pool, I turned the Humanist Society book face down on a poolside table, convinced it held no answers. I felt I had tried religion, and it too had failed me. At that exact moment, I heard the *clank* of our backyard's chain-link fence gate. I will never forget that sound.

It was my sister-in-law Jackie and my brother Edwin entering the yard. Jackie had recently become deeply religious, and we had often debated her stories of healings and answered prayers. "Show me the x-rays," I'd say. "Show me the lab results. Then I'll believe." Jackie was undeterred. That day, instead of another story, she handed me a book called *A New Song* by Pat Boone.

I laughed inwardly. *Pat Boone? Really?* I thought he was the biggest hypocrite alive—too "perfect," too pious, too squeaky-clean in his white buckskin shoes.

That night, I opened the book, expecting to be annoyed. But in the preface Boone wrote something that startled me: "This book contains things I wouldn't want my daughters to read."

Suddenly, I was intrigued. *What in the world has Pat Boone been up to?*

Boone shared how fame had taken him from church to Hollywood to Las Vegas—and how his marriage was on the verge of collapse. That's when his wife invited a man named George Otis to their home. Otis was president of the Lear Jet Corporation, a man Boone respected. Otis had undergone a powerful spiritual experience as part of the Charismatic Movement.

Otis told Boone that what he lacked was the Holy Spirit and offered to pray for him to receive it. Boone agreed. Otis laid hands on him, prayed, and announced, "Now you can speak in tongues." Boone tried but no words came forth. Otis disappeared into a back room to pray. He returned minutes later and said, "God has shown me that you have the gift of tongues—but you are not to verbalize; instead, you are to sing what will be your new song."

Boone opened his mouth and was able to sing in a language he didn't know.

Reading that, I was stunned. *If I were God,* I thought, *that's exactly how I would do it—I'd want Boone to sing with his beautiful baritone voice, in tongues, a language he didn't know*.

It was two o'clock in the morning when I put the book down. Something had shifted inside me. For the first time, faith had translated into my heart.

And then, I felt a Presence at the end of my bed. I don't know if it was God, Jesus, or an angel. But it was real. I heard, "I want you to have the gift of the Holy Spirit, but it is up to you."

I responded, "Lord, I want everything You have for me."

In that moment, I felt as though God was pouring liquid love through the top of my head into every part of my being. The love I felt was a thousand times more powerful than anything I had ever experienced. In my heart of hearts, for the first time in my life I knew that God was real. I also knew that I knew that I knew that God had known me from the beginning of creation. This moment had always been waiting for me, just as it is for every person on earth.

When I awoke the next morning, the feeling hadn't faded. I was beaming. My salivary glands were involuntarily releasing fluid when I opened my mouth. As an ENT specialist, I knew salivation was controlled by the autonomic nervous system. I couldn't do this on my own. It was as if God had filled every fiber of my being with his love.

At church that morning, a man approached me and asked, "John, what happened to you? You're aglow."

I smiled and said, "The Holy Spirit has come into my life."

He looked startled, turned, and hurriedly ran in the other direction.

That is the story of my spiritual awakening.

I cannot explain everything that happened, but I know it was real, authentic. It changed every aspect of my life. That empty place inside me was filled. Not with religion. Not with philosophy. Not even with good works. It was filled with a Presence—with divine love that had always known me.

This isn't a prescription for others. It's simply a story. My story. I share it now because perhaps, somewhere, someone else may be sitting by their own swimming pool, turning over the last page of another book, wondering if this is all there is to life.

Encounter Two: The Call to Become a Plastic Surgeon

After my encounter with God's overwhelming love, everything in my life changed. I was filled with a joy that spilled into every part of my being. I continued my work as an Ear, Nose, and Throat (ENT) physician and began an early Monday morning physician Bible study at the hospital. Ten to twelve doctors joined me regularly. But one morning, no one came. I decided to wait alone and read Scripture anyway.

I opened my Bible randomly and found myself reading from the book of Hosea. I was astonished to see God commanding the prophet Hosea: *"Take unto yourself an adulterous woman and children of unfaithfulness because the land is guilty of the vilest adultery in departing from the Lord"* (Hosea 1:2–3). In chapter 3, I read: *"Love her as the Lord loves the Israelites, though they turn to other gods and love the sacred raisin cakes"* (Hosea 3:1).

I was stunned. Why would God ask a prophet to *live* the message rather than just *deliver* it? Then I heard, with inward authority: **"I am calling you into plastic surgery. In plastic surgery, you will see lesions and blemishes on people and be trained to take care of them."**

In that moment, I felt as if a coin turned over and I viewed the other side, and I heard: **"And by My Spirit, I will show you lesions and blemishes on My church, and you will know how to take care of those as well."**

Like Hosea, I felt I was being asked to live the message God had for His people.

I was stunned. Why me? Why plastic surgery? As an ENT specialist, I had been trained in nasal surgery and loved performing rhinoplasties. But to follow this call meant I would have to abandon my established medical practice, move from Shreveport (which had no plastic surgery residency program), and sell the beautiful Tudor home Pat and I loved. That evening, I told her everything. Shocked, Pat urged me to confirm the call with the men in our weekly prayer group.

When I shared it, the men were surprised but sensed the call might be genuine. Still, I fasted and prayed for days, asking for clarity. Finally, I gave God a condition: **"Lord, if You are truly calling me into plastic surgery, there's only one man I want to train under—Dr. Ralph Millard in Miami. If You're the Creator of the universe and if You are truly calling me into plastic surgery, You can make that happen."**

Millard had authored, *The Principles & Art of Plastic Surgery*, as well as the encyclopedic three-volume textbook entitled: *Cleft Craft: The Evolution of Its Surgery*. Millard had created the techniques used by most plastic surgeons for repair of cleft lip and palate deformities. His commanding presence at plastic surgery conventions had made him the most well-known, respected, and in many ways the most feared plastic surgeon in the world.

My exposure to the brilliance of Millard happened a decade before while I was an Ear, Nose, & Throat resident-in-training. A 33-year-old man arrived in our clinic with a mastoid infection which I treated. He also had a cleft lip that had never been repaired. I asked if he was interested in having his lip repaired and he agreed with enthusiasm. There was no plastic surgery residency program in our hospital, so I went to the library and found an article by Ralph Millard which showed step-by-step precisely how to repair a cleft lip.

A few days later, in the operating room, I followed Millard's directions and post-operatively the man's lip looked perfect. I was captivated by Millard's ability to write an article so well that I could execute a cleft lip operation though I had never seen one done. Thereafter, every month I looked in plastic surgery journals for anything written by Ralph Millard. Little did I know at the time that ten years later Millard would figure so prominently in my life.

A Door Opens

Having "challenged" God to open a door for me to train under Ralph Millard, I wrote Millard to inquire about being a resident in his plastic surgery program. Weeks later, Pat and I flew to Miami. At his office, Millard informed me he had no openings for three years and advised me to find another residency. He said after my training was complete, I could come and do a Fellowship with him. Before walking out, Millard verbalized aloud so I could hear what he wrote across the top of my letter: "This man can have the first residency opening that becomes available."

It was both encouraging and discouraging. When I called the American Society of Plastic Surgeons, I was told, "Every program in America is full. There are no openings." This made me think I had only imagined God was calling me to be a plastic surgeon.

The more I researched the process, I found even more hurdles:

- There was no residency opening in Millard's program for three years
- There was no opening in any plastic surgery residency program in the U.S.
- I did not have a Florida medical license
- Florida didn't accept other states' medical licenses by reciprocity
- I had not completed a four-year General Surgery residency, a requirement
- I was a board-certified Otolaryngologist (ENT), but not a General Surgeon.

I told God: **"If You've called me, You will have to overcome these hurdles."**

A Step of Faith

Despite opposition from fellow Christians who said God calls people to be a missionary, not a plastic surgeon, I could not deny what I had heard.

With Pat's support, I decided to take a step of faith. We put our home up for sale, packed up our five children and her mother who lived with us, and drove to Miami. We found a home for lease in Key Biscayne. The following Friday, I showed up at Millard's office with no appointment. He didn't seem to be happy with me and asked: "What are you doing here? I told you to go find a residency somewhere else and later you could come here for a Fellowship."

I explained there were no residency openings and that I wanted to be in plastic surgery and train under him, even if that meant I had to wait years for an opening. Millard stared at me and then said, "I have a residency position for you. It will only be for six months, but I will find a spot after that so you can complete your training." I was elated. I felt God had opened a residency for me in one of the most prestigious plastic surgery programs in the country.

Millard then said, "John, you better rush home, get packed, and return quickly because I only have six-months to work with you. We don't want to waste a moment."

I said I would rush back but didn't tell Dr. Millard we were already unpacked and settled in a house on Key Biscayne.

Every Obstacle Falls

On Monday morning, I joined Millard's Grand Rounds. I told the senior resident, Tony Wolfe, that I was concerned because I didn't have a Florida medical license. He shrugged: "Florida won't give a resident-in-training a license. They don't want you staying in Florida after you complete your residency. You don't need a Florida license."

Blocks #3 and 4 – cleared.

I then said that I have another problem: "I am an otolaryngologist, not a General Surgeon." Tony said, "Now, that's a problem." A few moments later, Millard walked in and seeing me he smiled and said, "This man moves too fast even for me." Then he announced to everyone: "Last week, the board voted to accept surgical sub-specialists. John will be the first ENT man we've ever taken as a resident."

Blocks #5 and 6 – cleared.

Millard never even asked about my medical license or training background. And somehow, he had space for me when all programs were said to be filled in America. It was a magnificent experience training with Dr. Millard, observing a great surgeon provide the best care possible for his patients.

Blocks #1 and 2 – cleared.

God's Provision

When my six months was ending with Millard, he was able to place me in a great follow-up residency in Norfolk, Virginia where I trained under Dr. Charlie Horton who was the current President of the American Society of Plastic Surgeons. His colleagues were all exceptional. I completed my training and returned home to Shreveport.

The first thing I did after returning home was to commit to weeks of prayer and fasting to hear what God wanted me to do—only to receive dead silence from God. This left me discouraged and thinner by 20 pounds. When I shared my disappointment with Pat, with all her wisdom and love she said, "Maybe you are supposed to go to work."

So, I did. I joined two other plastic surgeons in Shreveport and began doing exactly what God had said I would do: treating lesions and blemishes—external and, eventually, the internal. Over time, I opened my own private practice and continued to grow as a board-certified plastic and reconstructive surgeon.

Encounter Three: The Call to Priesthood

For many years, I served faithfully as a plastic surgeon in Shreveport. Day after day, my mornings began with the same prayer: "Lord, is this the day You are calling me full-time into ministry?" I couldn't shake the sense that God had more for me to do. But what did that mean? Was I being called to medical missions? Or was it something entirely different—perhaps pastoral ministry?

Whenever I shared these stirrings with Pat, she would remind me of the good work I was already doing, like using my training in microsurgery to replant the totally amputated arm of four-year-old Robert or restoring little Chad's face after a devastating shotgun blast. She was right—I was doing meaningful, and at times almost miraculous work to help people in their hour of great need. But deep down, I still felt a divine nudge, a whisper I couldn't ignore.

For fifteen years, I prayed for clarity. And for fifteen years, silence. Eventually, I wondered if I had misunderstood altogether. Perhaps God had never called me to anything beyond the fulfilling work I was already doing as a plastic surgeon. Maybe this was enough.

An Unsettling Invitation

At the time, Pat and I owned a beautiful building we used as a day surgery center with three operating rooms. We dedicated the facility to the Lord and prayed that God would send the patients that God wanted us to serve. Over many years, we restored the facility, room by room, and gave thanks for what we believed to be a beautiful gift to God (and from God).

One day, my receptionist said a man had arrived and wanted to see me. I met him in the lobby as he was clearly marveling at the beauty of our facility. He said, "Dr. Graham, this would make the perfect building for a drug and alcohol rehabilitation center."

I politely declined. As I walked back to my office, an unspoken prejudice surfaced in my mind: *I don't want a bunch of addicts and winos tearing up our place.* It clearly wasn't my best moment.

A month passed, and a second man came to me with the same idea. Again, I said no. And the following month, yet another man arrived with the same request. For the third time, I said no. But this time, as I walked back to my office, I heard an inner voice that cut me to my core: **"It is interesting you do not want your building used for drug and alcohol rehabilitation when alcohol has beset your family for four generations."**

I froze. It was the exact opposite of what I had been thinking. And I *knew* it was God speaking to me. I remembered our dedication prayer—how we had asked God to send those He wanted us to serve in our building. And now, not one but three messengers had come offering a new and different use for our facility. God was answering my fifteen-year prayer—but I had been too focused on preserving our beloved building to even recognize He was speaking. I was convicted and prayed: "Father, forgive me. Everything I have belongs to You—including this building and my medical practice. Now, I hear You asking me to lay it down and I will."

Laying It Down

Closing my practice was the hardest decision of my professional life. I took fifteen years' worth of patient charts and placed them on the shelves in another plastic surgeon's office. Each name stirred memories, and my heart ached as I entrusted their care to someone else. I had loved being a physician. It had never been just a job for me. But I couldn't deny God's call. God was asking for more.

We leased the building and packed our lives into boxes. Pat and I, with hearts open but uncertain, headed first to Fuller Theological Seminary in Pasadena, California, and later to the Episcopal Theological Seminary of the Southwest in Austin, Texas.

I was finally stepping into the full-time ministry that I had prayed about for over so many years.

The Awakening of a New Vision

What I discovered in seminary reshaped me. My years at Fuller and then in Austin were transformative—emotionally, intellectually, and spiritually. I came to understand the Bible not as a set of literal word-for-word dictations from God, but as a sacred unfolding of divine revelation, spoken through inspired men across centuries.

And the pinnacle of that revelation was Jesus—the Word made flesh. In Him, I saw not the wrath of God, but the **boundless, inclusive love** of a God who embraces all people, of every faith, in every condition, and in every place throughout human history. That realization didn't diminish my childhood faith; it fulfilled it. Even as a child I had always sensed God's love and not God's wrath. Now, I saw it with theological clarity. And that love opened in me a new joy, a new purpose.

Preparation for the Path Ahead

The call to priesthood didn't erase my identity as a physician—it built upon it. Seminary was not an escape from medicine but what I saw as a divine pivot. It was a time of preparation. I would soon find myself at the intersection of faith and science, called into the ministry of healing—not just of bodies, but of hearts, minds, and communities.

And so, I stepped into the priesthood—called not only to serve the Church, but to help bridge two seemingly distant worlds: the spiritual and the scientific. In time, that calling would lead me to assume leadership of an institute where both could thrive together.

Encounter Four: Uniting Science and Spirituality

I had no idea that such a place existed. An institute within the Texas Medical Center—one of the largest and most advanced medical complexes in the world—dedicated not only to technology or surgery, but to the sacred meeting of science and the spirit.

The Institute for Spirituality and Health, once known as the Institute of Religion, was founded in 1955 with a bold and visionary purpose: to explore the healing connection between body, mind, and soul. Its first director, the Rev. Dawson Bryan, helped pioneer the concept of hospital chaplaincy—clergy serving within medical institutions as companions of comfort and faith.

Years later, while a priest at St. Martin's Episcopal Church, I found myself sitting on the board of the Institute for Spirituality and Health, not yet realizing that it would one day become the place where the many threads of my life would be drawn together into one.

A Door Opens, Again

In 2009, I was required to retire from full-time parish ministry. Seventy-two is the age of mandatory retirement in the Episcopal Church, but—I didn't feel finished. Not inwardly.

I began serving as a pastoral counselor at a rehabilitation center for those suffering from addiction. Recalling God's reminder that alcohol had beset my family for four generations. Honored to witness broken lives begin to mend. But quietly, I sensed that something else—something more—was stirring.

Then, in the spring of 2010, I received the invitation from the chairman of the Institute for Spirituality and Health's Board of Trustees: "Would you consider becoming President of the Institute?"

It took my breath away.

Here was a place committed to integrating the very two worlds I had lived in—medicine and spirituality. Surgery and sacrament. Hospital and sanctuary. I didn't plan it. I couldn't have. But I knew in the marrow of my bones: God had.

A Calling Revealed

When I left medicine and entered seminary, I had no knowledge that such an Institute even existed. Now, decades later, I was being invited to lead it. I had trained as a physician under Ralph Millard. I had stood at hospital bedsides, scrubbed in for operations, felt the tension of life and death in my hands. Later, I had stood at altars, offered prayers, baptized infants, celebrated marriages, and walked with the grieving.

Now, finally, both paths converged. Medicine and religion; science and spirituality.

It felt like—no, it *was*—divine orchestration. A design too intricate and complex to be my own. This was not coincidence. It was a calling. This was my destiny. The place I had been unknowingly moving toward my entire life.

Each morning as President of the Institute, I awoke with joy. I had lived both callings—in the body and in the spirit—and now was invited to help build something that honored both. And to offer a small step toward healing a division that had persisted for too long. Medicine and faith.

Mission Accomplished—The Institute Renewed

Over the next twelve years, the Institute entered a season of renewed growth. With generous support, we able to expand our staff, launch new programs, and forge partnerships with other organizations that deepened our mission.

A humorous moment greeted me soon after I arrived at ISH. I was halfway through hanging my framed certificates on my new office wall when our secretary walked in and asked, "What are you doing?" I replied, "I'm putting my plaques on the wall." She paused and said, "Why are you doing that?" I smiled and said, "Because I intend to stay." And stay I did—for more than twelve years, the longest tenure of any President in the Institute's then fifty-five-year history. It felt like destiny, as though every step in my journey—first as physician, then as priest—had been leading me to this place. At ISH, everything converged, and I found a deep joy in the work.

My time at ISH was about connecting with people and building relationships—within our board, with foundation chairs, with academic professors, and with the community of people in healthcare providers and chaplains of Houston hospitals. Relationships built trust and trust provided the resources we needed to establish ISH in the Texas Medical Center. I have deep gratitude for a wonderful staff of co-workers, for this has always been a team effort and not my work alone. It was the experience of working together with so many beautiful, talented people that made it such a joy to serve as President and CEO of ISH.

Where I Am Now

I served for just over twelve years at the Institute and am blessed knowing, with God's help, the Institute has grown in every way and is financially secure. Upon my retirement, Stuart Nelson was selected by the Institute's board to become its next President and CEO. I now serve as President Emeritus and coordinate the work of our adjunct faculty and continue my weekly bereavement support group meetings—a sacred space of shared sorrow and healing.

In retirement, I have been able to complete a research project, write and defend my dissertation, and receive a Ph.D. degree in Mind-Body Medicine with specialization in Psychophysiology. I've also been gifted with time to reflect, to write, and to gather the many threads of this journey into the book you now hold.

What I have shared is not a theological argument, but a story. A human story. A journey from certainty to mystery, from exclusion to embrace, from doctrine to love. And at the heart of it, I now know this: **God is love. And love is never limited to those who think alike.**

Invitation to Encounter Five

At the beginning of these Four Encounters I said if you wished to continue our journey together that I would tell you how that can happen. I'm sure you'll agree, the journey of life is always a mystery. I do not know which doors will open and which will close. God knows, not me. Yet, I have found the journey to be filled with surprise, joy, and lament. The journey can also bring together that which divides people into separate camps: the division between science and spirituality being but one example. We are all too aware of division and conflict within relationships, organizations, and among nations. If you are interested in being part of a journey that seeks unity, peace, and mutual love, I invite you to join me and explore together God's next Encounter at: **www.johnkgraham.com**.

About the Author

John K. Graham, M.D., Ph.D., D.Min. has served as a physician, an Episcopal priest, and as President/CEO of the Institute for Spirituality and Health at the Texas Medical Center (ISH). Graham received his M.D. degree from Tulane Medical School in New Orleans, was board certified in two medical specialties, and has a Ph.D. in Mind-Body Medicine with specialization in Psychophysiology.

Dr. Graham received national media exposure in 1977 when he used microsurgery to successfully replant the totally amputated arm of a 4-year-old boy. The event was widely publicized, and John and the boy appeared together on several national television programs.

In 1990, John responded to God's call to attend seminary and received a Master of Divinity degree from the Episcopal Theological Seminary of the Southwest in Austin. In 2001, he received a Doctor of Ministry degree in Group Development from Seabury-Western Theological Seminary in Evanston, Illinois.

Following his ordination, John served as an Episcopal priest at St. Matthew's Episcopal Church in Austin, Trinity Episcopal Church in Houston, and, for twelve years was an Associate Rector at St. Martin's Episcopal Church, in Houston.

John was a founding member of the Board of Directors of St. Luke's Episcopal Health Charities, a ministry to the medically underserved. He also served for 9 years as a member of the board of directors of LifeGift Houston, an organization providing life-giving organ and tissue transplantation for individuals, many who were otherwise at the point of death

In 2001, Dr. Graham completed a two-year Fellowship in Psychotherapy at the Houston-Galveston Psychoanalytic Institute. He has served as a counselor at the Inter-Face Samaritan Counseling Center in Houston and as Spiritual Director for the staff.

In March of 2010, John was elected President and Chief Executive Officer of the Institute for Spirituality and Health (ISH), in Houston. For 70 years, the Institute has promoted complementary and integrative healthcare to students in training at five medical and nursing schools in Houston and Galveston, Texas.

John served as President/CEO for 12 years, until June 30, 2022. He is now President Emeritus and serves part-time at ISH where he coordinates the activities of a coalition of Adjunct Faculty and facilitates a weekly on-line bereavement support group.

John and his wife, Pat, have five adult children and many grandchildren. Recently, he completed a program through Harvard Medical School entitled, "AI in Medicine."

Contact John at his website: www.johnkgraham.com.

References Cited

Achtner, W. (n.d.) Time, eternity and trinity [SR21.physics.auth.gr], Berlin, GR *Times*. 1-18. https://sr21.physics.auth.gr/Times/Dialogue/Achtner_final.pdf

Alter, M. G. (1994). *Resurrection Psychology: An Understanding of Human Personality Based on the Life and Teachings of Jesus*. Eugene, OR: Wiph & Stock Publishers, 71.

Alexander, E., III (2012). *Proof of Heaven: A Neurosurgeon's Journey into the Afterlife*. New York, NY: Simeon & Schuster.

Alexander, E., III (2021). The revelations of primordial consciousness. In, *The Mysteries of Reality: Dialogues with Visionary Scientists*, Gayle Kimball [Ed.], Alresford, Hampshire, UK: John Hunt Publishing, 31-58.

Angel H. F., Seitz R. J. (2024). Credition and the neurobiology of belief: the brain function in believing. *Academia Biology* 2024; 2. https://doi.org/10.20935/AcadBiol7359

Ano, G. G. & Pargament, K. I. (2013). Predictors of spiritual struggles: An exploratory study. *Mental Health, Religion, & Culture*, 16(4), 419-434. http://dx.doi.org/10.1080/13674676.2012.680434

Balboni, T. A., Vander-Wheele, T. J., Doan-Soares, D. D., Long, K. N. G., Ferrell, B. R., Fitchett, G., Koenig, H. G., Bain, Paul A., Puchalski, C., Steinhauser, K. E., & Sulmasy D. P. . (2022). Spirituality in serious illness and health. *JAMA*, 328(2), 184-197. https://doi.org/10.1001/jama/2022.11086

Baron-Cohen, S. (2011). *The Science of Evil: On Empathy and the Origins of Cruelty*. New York, NY: Basic Books.

Bassett, J. F. (2014, May 27). Fears of finitude and eternity: Attitudes about immortality and the afterlife in selected movies. *Studies in Popular Culture, Spring 36*(2), 67-82, www.pcasacas.org.

Benson, H. (1996). *Timeless Healing: The Power and Biology of Belief.* New York, NY: Simon & Schuster. 49-95.

Bergman, J. (2017). Why the Miller-Urey research proves biblical creation. *Apologiaway1.wordpress.com.* https://apologiaway1.wordpress.com/2017/01/01/why-the-miller-urey-experiment-proves-biblical-creation/

Bongard, J. and Levin, M. (2021). Living things are not (20th century) machines: Updating mechanism metaphors in light of the modern science of machine behavior. *Frontiers in Ecology and Evolution, 9* | Article 650726, 1-15. https://doi.org/10.3389/fevo.2021.

Braden, G. (2025). *Pure Human: The Hidden Truth of Our Divinity, Power, and Destiny*. New York, NY: Hay House. 151-152

Briggs, J. & Peat, F. D. (1999). *Seven Life Lessons of Chaos: Spiritual Wisdom from the Science of Change*. New York, NY: Harper-Collins Publishers.

Carter, E. C. (2020). D. A. Leeming (ed.), *Encyclopedia of Psychology and Religion*. https://doi.org/10.1007/978-3-030-24348-7

Cave, S. (2012). *Immortality: The Quest to Live Forever and How It Drives Civilization*. New York, NY: Random House.

Chestney, K. (2024). *The Illumination Code: 7 Keys to Unlock Your Quantum Intelligence*. Novato, CA: New World Library.

Chopra, D. (2015). *Quantum Healing: Exploring the Frontiers of Mind/Body Medicine*. New York: Bantum Books, Random House Publishing Co., 278-279.

Craig, W. L., (2001). God, time, and eternity: The coherence of theism II: Eternity. Springer Science Business Media Dordrecht. https://dio.org/10.1007/978-94-017-1715-1

Crick, F. & Koch, C. (1990). Towards a neurobiological theory of consciousness. in *Seminars in the Neurosciences, 2*, 263–275.

Curlin, F. A. , Sellergren, S. A., & Lantos, J. D. (2007). Physicians' observations and interpretation of the influence of religion and spirituality on health. *Arch internal Medicine, 167*(7), 649-654. https://doi.org/10.1001/archinte.167.7.649

Currivan, J. (2017). *The Cosmic Hologram: In-formation at the Center of Creation*. Rochester, Vermont: Inner Traditions/Bear & Company. Kindle Editon.

Davidson, M. (2017). Vaccination as a cause of autism—myths and controversies. *Dialogues in clinical neuroscience, 19*(4), 403-407.

Davies, P. (2000). *The Fifth Miracle: The Search for the Origin and Meaning of Life*. New York: Simon & Schuster.

De Florio, C. & Frigerio, A. (2013). God, evil, and Alvin Plantinga on the free-will defense. *European J of Philosophy of Religion, 5*(3), 75-94.

Denton, M. (2020). *The Miracle of the Cell*. Seattle: Discovery Institute Press.

Diamond, E. F. (2008). Miracles. *The Linacre Quarterly,* 75:4, 345-351, https://doi.org/10.1179/002436308803889413

Doncel, M. G., S. J. (2004). The kenosis of the creator and of the created co-creator. *Zygon 39*(4), 791-800.

Egnor, M. (2023). Neuroscience and dualism. In: *Minding the Brain: Models of the Mind, Information, Empirical Science*. Angus J. Menuge, Brian R. Krouse, & Robert J. Marks [Eds.]. Seattle, WA: Discovery Institute Press.

Egnor, M. & O'Leary, D. (2025). *The Immortal Mind: A Neurosurgeon's Case for the Existence of the Soul*. Hachette Nashville. Kindle Edition, p. 6-8.

Emoto, M. (2007). *The Miracle of Water*. New York, NY: Atria Books.

Faggin, Federico (2024). *Irreducible: Consciousness, Life, Computers, and Human Nature*. Alresford Hampshire, UK: John Hunt Publishing. p.39.

Feynman, R. P. (1955, December). The value of science: of all its many values, the greatest must be the freedom to doubt. *Engineering and Science, XIX*, 13-15.

Frank, D. L., Khorshid, L., Kiffer, J. F., Moravec, C. S., & McKee, M. G. (2010). Biofeedback in medicine: Who, when, why, and how? *Mental Health in Family Medicine, 7*, 85-91.

Gabriel, R. (2021). Affect, belief, and the arts. *Frontiers in Psychology, 12*[Article 757234] 1-16.

Gupta, M. (2025, Jan 20). Why AI Agents will be a huge disaster. Medium. *Data Science in Your Pocket*. https://medium.com/data-science-in-your-pocket/why-ai-agents-will-be-a-huge-disaster-9a68d9db18a1

Hagen, R. L. (1997). In Praise of the Null Hypothesis Statistical Test. *American Psychologist, 52*(1), 15-24.

Harris, W. S., Gowda, M., Kolb, J. W., Strychacz, C. P., Vacek, J. L., Jones, P. G., Forker, A., O'Keefe, J. H., & McCallister, B. D. (Oct. 25, 1999). A randomized, controlled trial of the effects of remote, intercessory prayer on outcomes in patients admitted to the coronary care unit. *Arch Internal Medicine 159*, 2273-2278.

Hawking, S. W. (1988). *A Brief History of Time*. New York, NY: Bantam Books.

Hawkins, D. R. (2012). *Power vs. Force: The Hidden Determinants of Human Behavior*. New York, NY: Hay House, Inc.

HeartMath Institute (Downloaded April 4, 2025). *Science of the heart*. https://www.heartmath.org/research/science-of-the-heart/

Hotez, P. (2019). America and Europe's new normal: the return of vaccine-preventable diseases. *Pediatric Research, 85*, 912–914. https://doi.org/10.1038/s41390-019-0354-3, and www.nature.com/articles/s41390-019-0354-3

Hume D. (1993). *An Enquiry Concerning Human Understanding, and Other Writings*. (2nd Ed. by Eric Steinberg), Indianapolis: Hackett Publishing Co.

Ikerd, J. (2007). Science and the sacred. In, *Science, Religion, and Society: An Encyclopedia of History, Culture, and Controversy*. Vol. 2., Arri Eisen & Gary Laderman [Eds.]. Armonk, NY: M. E. Sharpe publisher. 499-506.

James, W. (1889). *The psychology of belief, In Literature and Philosophy in Nineteenth Century British Culture* (p29-36). Routledge.

Jimenez, M., Prieto, A., Hinojosa, J. A., & Montoro, P. R. (2025). Consciousness under the spotlight: The problem of measuring subjective experience. *Wiley Interdisciplinary Reviews: Cognitive Science* [16:e1697]. https://doi.org/10.1002/2cs.1697

Jung, C. G. (2009). *The Red Book: A Reader's Edition* (Ed., Sonu Shamdasani). New York, NY: W. W. Norton & Co.

Kimball, G. (2021). *The Mysteries of Reality: Dialogues with Visionary Scientists*. John Hunt Publishing Ltd., Alresford, Hampshire, UK.

Kokubo, H., Nemoto, Y. & Kawano, K. (2017). Discussion on methodology of water crystal formation as a detection system for PSI. *Journal of Parapsychology, 81*(1), 73-86.

Koenig, H. G., Vanderweele, T. J., & Peteet, J. R. (2023). *Handbook of Religion and Health, 4th Ed.* New York, NY: Oxford University Press.

Kripal, J. J., Anzali, A., Jain, A. R., Prophet, E., & Sanchez, S. (2024). *Comparing Religions: The Study of Us that Changes Us, (2nd Ed.)*. Hoboken, NJ: Wiley-Blackwell Publishing.

Krohn, E. G. & Kripal, J. J. (2018). *Changed in a Flash: One woman's Near-Death Experience and Why a Scholar Thinks it Empowers us All*. Berkley, CA: North Atlantic Books.

Laszlo, E. (2004, 2nd Ed. 2007). *Science and the Akashic Field: An Integral Theory of Everything*. Rochester, Vermont: Inner Traditions.

Laszlo, E. (2017). *The Intelligence of the Cosmos: Why are we here? New answers from the frontiers of science*. Rochester, Vermont: Inner Traditions.

Laszlo, E. (2020). *Reconnecting to the Source: The new science of spiritual experience. How it can change you, and How it can transform the world*. New York: St. Martin's Press.

Lewis, C. S. (1947). *Miracles*. New York: HarperCollins.

Levin, M. (2022). Biology, life, aliens, evolution, embryogenesis & xenobots. *YouTube: Lex Fridman Podcast # 325*. https://www.youtube.com/watch?v=p3lsYlod5OU&t=60s

Lopez-Martinez, A., Serrano-Ibanez, E. R., Ruiz-Parraga, G. T., Gomez-Perez, L., Ramirez-Maestre, C., & Esteve, R. (2018). Physical health consequences of interpersonal trauma: A systematic review of the role of psychological variables. *Trauma, Violence & Abuse, 19*(3), 305-322.

Lothane, Z. (2007). The power of spoken word in life, psychiatry, and psychoanalysis: A contribution to interpersonal psychoanalysis. *American Journal of Psychoanalysis, 67*, 260-274.

Mandl, K. D. (2025). How AI could reshape health care – rise in direct-to-consumer models. *JAMA, 333*(19), 1667-1669.

McCraty, R. & Zayas, M. A. (2014). Cardiac coherence, self-regulation, autonomic stability, and psychosocial well-being. *Frontiers in Psychology 5*[Article 1090], 1-13.

McCraty, R. (April 4, 2025). *Heart-brain neurodynamics: The making of Emotions*. HeartMath Institute. https://www.heartmath.org/assets/uploads/2015/03/heart-brain-neurodyamics.pdf

Menuge, A. J. L. (2023). Declining physicalism and resurgent alternatives. In: *Minding the Brain: Models of the Mind, Information, Empirical Science*. Angus J. L. Menuge, Brian R. Krouse, & Robert J. Marks [Eds.]. Seattle, WA: Discovery Institute Press, 37-78.

Meijer, D. K. F. (2012). The information universe: On the missing link in concepts of the architecture of reality. *Syntropy 1*, 1-64.

Meyer, S. C. (2021). *Return of the God Hypothesis: Three Scientific Discoveries That Reveal the Mind Behind the Universe*. New York, NY: HarperCollins Publisher, 289-298, 436-439.

Miller, L. (2014). Neuroanatomical correlates of religiosity and spirituality: A study in adults at high and low familiar risk for depression. *JAMA Psychiatry, 71*(2), 128-135. https://doi.org/10.1001/jamapsychiatry.2013.3067

Miller, L., Balodis, I. M., McClintock, C. H., Xu, J., Lacadie, C. M., Sinha, R. & Potenza, M. N. (2019). Neural correlates of personalized spiritual experiences. *Cerebral Cortex, 29*, 2331-2338. https://doi.org/10.1093/cercor/bhy102

Miller, L. (2012). Introduction, *The Oxford Handbook of Psychology and Spirituality*. New York, NY: Oxford University Press. 1-6.

Miller, L. (2015). *The Spiritual Child: The New Science on Parenting for Health and Lifelong Thriving*. New York, NY: St. Martin's Press.

Miller, L. (2021). *The Awakened Brain: The New Science of Spirituality and our Quest for an Inspired Life*. New York, NY: Random House.

Miller, S. L. (1953). A Production of Amino Acids Under Possible Primitive Earth Conditions. *Science, 117*, 528-529.

Miller, W. R. & Thoresen, C. E. (2003). Spirituality, religion, and health: An emerging research field. *American Psychologist, 58*(1), 24-35. http://doi.org/10.1037/0003-066X.58.1.24

Modell, H., Cliff, W., Michael, J., McFarland, J., Wenderoth, M. P., & Wright, A. (2015). *Advances in Physiological Education, 39*(4), 259-266.

Moss, D. (1998). Biofeedback, mind-body medicine, and the higher limits of human nature. *Humanistic and transpersonal psychology: A historical and biographical sourcebook*, 145-161.

Newberg, A. B. (2006). *Why We Believe What We Believe*. New York: Simon & Schuster, 3-4.

Oboli, V. N. (2025, June 3). A stinging slap. *JAMA, 333*(21), 1870-1871. https://doi.org/10.1001/jama.2025.4

Olive, J. K., Hotez, P. J., Damania, A., Nolan, M. S. (2018) The state of the antivaccine movement in the United States: A focused examination of nonmedical exemptions in states and counties. *PLoS Med 15*(6): e1002578. https://doi.org/10.1371/journal.pmed.1002578

O'Shea-Brown, G. (2021). *Healing Complex Posttraumatic Stress Disorder: A Clinician's Guide*. New York, NY: Springer.

Padgett, Jason (retrieved 2025, May 6). You are the movie the universe is watching. *Facebook.com/Videos.* https://www.facebook.com/100063489523265/videos/10260782707399

Pargament, K. I., Smith, B. W., Koenig, H. G., & Perez, L. (1998). Patterns of positive and negative religious coping with major life stressors. *Journal for the Scientific Study of Religion, 37*, 710–724.

Pargament, K., Magya-Russell, G. M., & Murray-Swank, N. A. (2005). The sacred and the search for significance: Religion as a unique process. *Journal of Social Issues, 61*(4), 665-687.

Parker, E. T., Cleaves, J. H., Burton, A. S., Glavin, D. P., Dworkin, J. P., Zhou, M., Bada, J. L., Fernández, F. M. (2014). Conducting Miller-Urey Experiments. *J. Vis. Exp*. (83), e51039, https://doi.org10.3791/51039

Pastis, S. (2025, May 3). Pearls Before Swine. New York, NY: Hearst Publishing: *Houston Chronicle*, p. A-10.

Pastwa-Wojciechowska, B., Grzegorzewska, I., & Wojciechowska, A. (2021). The role of religious values and beliefs in shaping mental health and disorders. *Religions 12*: 840. https://doi.org/10.3390/rel12100840

Pennycook, G., Cheyne, J. A, Koehler, D. J., & Fugelsang, J. A. (2020). On the belief that beliefs should change according to evidence: Implications for conspiratorial, moral, paranormal, political, religious, and science beliefs. *Judgment and Decision Making,15*(4), 476–498.

Peters, Ted (2019). The science of evil and the theology of evil. *Theology and Science, 17*(3), 297-304. https://doi.org/10.1080/14746700.2019.1632518

Pew Research Center (December 7, 2023). Spirituality among Americans. https://www.pewresearch.org/religion/2023/12/07/spirituality-among-americans/.

Plantinga, A. (1989). *God, Freedom, and Evil*. Grand Rapids, MI: Wm. B. Eerdmans Publishing.

Polkinghorne, J. (2007). Integrating science and religion. In, *Science Religion, and Society: An Encyclopedia of History, Culture and Controversy*. Armonk, NY: M.E. Sharpe, Inc., p 7.

Porot, N. & Mandelbaum, E. (2020). The science of belief: A progress report. *WIREs Cognitive Science* [e1539], 1-17. https://doi.org/10.1002/wcs.1539

Prabhupada, A. C. (1983). *Bhagavad Gita as it is*. Los Angeles, CA: The Prabhupada Book Trust.

Prophet, M. L. & Prophet, E. C. (2004). *The Science of the Spoken Word*. Corwin Springs, MT: Summit University Press. xviii - xxi.

Rodriguez-Rosello, M. A. (2019). The holographic paradigm. *Documentos Y Articulos*. https://marosello.net/DOC/Main%20Menu/Universalism/The%20Holographic%20Paradigm.pdf

Rohr, R. (2016). *The Divine Dance: The Trinity and Your Transformation*. New Keningston, PA: Whitaker House Publishing, 61-69.

Rosmarin, D. H., Pirutinsky, S., Auerbach, R. P., Björgvinsson, T., Bigda-Peyton, J., Andersson, G., Pargament, K. I., & Krumrei, E. J. (2011). Incorporating spiritual beliefs into a cognitive model of worry. *Journal of Clinical Psychology, 67*, 691-700. https://doi.org/10.1002/jclp.20798

Ryder, G. (June 09, 2022). 7 miraculous stories about the power of healing prayers. *Readers Digest*. https://www.rd.com/list/prayers-for-healing/?utm_source=chatgpt.com

Sattin, D., Magnani, F. G., Bartesaghi, L., Caputo, M., Fitipaldo, A. B., Cacciatore, M., Picozzi, M., Leonardi, M. (2021). Theoretical models of consciousness: A scoping review. *Brain Sciences, 11*, 535. https://doi.org/10.3390/brainsci11050535

Schama, Simon (2006). *The Power of Art*. New York, NY: HarperCollins Publisher.

Schwartz, G. E. (2002). *The Afterlife Experiments: Breakthrough Scientific Evidence of Life After Death*. New York, NY: Atria Books, Simon & Schuster eBook.

Srivastava, J. N. (2011). *A Viable New Paradigm for Quantum Reality*. Hauppauge, New York: Nova Science Publishing.

Smee, S. (Nov. 16, 2018). "'At Eternity's Gate': A portrait of Vincent van Gogh as a tormented soul." *Washington Post*, [GALE |A562400014] (Accessed 28 Apr. 2025). Gale Academic https://gale.com/apps/doc/A562400014/AONE?u=anon~9218cb90&sid=googleScholar&xid=95bfd44e

Smith, David Livingstone (2024) *Less Than Human: Why We Demonize, Enslave, and Exterminate Others*. New York, NY: St. Martin's Press.

Spitzer, R. J., (2023). *Science at the Doorstep of God: Science and Reason in Support of God, the Soul, and Life After Death*. San Francisco, CA: Ignatius Press, 205-220.

Stroebe, M., Schut, H., & Stroebe, W. (2007). Health outcomes of bereavement. *Lancet, 370*, p1960-1973.

Succi, M. D., Chang, B. S., & Rao, A. S. (2025). Building the AI-enabled medical school of the future. *JAMA 333*(19), 1665-1666.

Swimme, B. T. & Tucker, M. E. (2011). *Journey of the Universe*. New Haven, CN: Yale University Press. 107-109.

Taghipour, M., Derakhshan, N., & Saffarian, A. (2019). At Eternity's Gate: Temporal lobe epilepsy and the genius of Vincent van Gogh. *Psychoiatria Danubina, 31*, 374-376. https://doi.org/10.24869/psyd.2019.374

Van Lommel, P., van Wees, R., Meyers, V., & Elfferich, I. (2001), Near-death experience in survivors of cardiac arrest: A prospective study in the Netherlands. *Lancet.358*. pp. 2039-2045. https://profezie3m.altervista.org/archivio/TheLancet_NDE.htm

Van Lommel, P. (2006). Near-death experience, consciousness, and the brain: A new concept about the continuity of our consciousness based on recent scientific research on near-death experience in survivors of cardiac arrest. *World Futures, 62*. 134-151. https://doi.org/10.1080/02604020500412808

Yaron, I., Melloni, L., Pitts, M., & Mudrik, L. (2021). The Consciousness Theories Studies (ConTraSt) database: Analyzing and comparing empirical studies of consciousness theories. *BioRxiv 06* [20.447863.2021]. https://doi.org/10.1101/2021.06.10.447863

Index

www.ingramcontent.com/pod-product-compliance
Lightning Source LLC
LaVergne TN
LVHW011517200926
848484LV00001B/54

* 9 7 9 8 2 9 5 4 6 6 6 8 7 *